Everything Egg Freezing

The Essential Step-By-Step Guide to Doing it Right

Brittany Hawkins & Catherine Hendy
Second Edition: March 2020

For our mothers, Brigid and Theresa,
and all the other women who made it ok to wait.

Acknowledgments

Thanks to the many women who graciously shared their personal stories and insights to sprinkle some "human" on top of the science in this book. Their names have been changed to respect their privacy. In addition, sincere thanks to our proofreader, John Hawkins, and everyone else who gave their valuable time and support in making this book happen: *Charl Burgess-Green, Ty Canning, Bailey DeWitt, Clare Dyson, Dr. Hamed Eltaher, Scarlett Edmiston, Gavin Aiken, Hollie Harrison, Ian Duvenage, Nina Elvin-Jensen, Karen Goldscher, Shannon Grant, Cecil Hendy, Theresa Hendy, Monica Ibanez, Susana Kennedy, Molly Kenward, Dr. Ola Khalil, Lauren Krasney, Jana Kruger, Emily Leung, Merilee McDougal, Brigid Mulligan, Rachel Naik, Jodi Neuhauser, Sharman Ordoyne, Alexandra Phelps, Aunnie Power, Chanél Roussou, Erika Wiese, and, of course, our "A team:" Adam and Arvind.*

Expert Panel and Advisory

We are indebted to our busy panel of experts for the time and knowledge they gave for this book, and for the incredible work they do helping women all over the world preserve their fertility:

- Professor Richard Anderson, BSc(Hons), PhD, MB. ChB, MRCOG, MD, CCST, FRCOG, FRC(Ed), Elsie Inglis Professor of Clinical Reproductive Science, Head of Section, Obstetrics and Gynaecology at the University of Edinburgh, Executive Committee of European Society of Human Reproduction and Embryology (ESHRE), Scientific and Clinical Advances Advisory Committee of the Human Fertilisation and Embryology Authority (HFEA)

- Dr. Diana E. Chavkin, MD, FACOG, Board Certified by ACOG in Obstetrics and Gynecology and Reproductive Endocrinology and Infertility, Fertility Physician at HRC Fertility, West Los Angeles

- Dr. Aimee Eyvazzadeh, MD, Board Certified Obstetrics and Gynecology, specializing in Reproductive Endocrinology and Infertility, Founder of eggwhisperer.com, San Ramon

- Dr. Carolyn Givens MD, Medical Co-Director, Pacific Fertility Center, San Francisco

- Dr. Eleni Greenwood Jaswa, MD, MSc, FACOG, Assistant Professor of Obstetrics, Gynecology and Reproductive Sciences at the University of California San Francisco

- Dr. Victor Hulme, MD, Gynecologist and Specialist in Reproductive Medicine, Aevitas Fertility Clinic, Cape Town, South Africa

- Valerie Landis, Fertility Patient Advocate, Egg Freezing and Cryopreservation Counselor, Founder of eggsperience.com + Eggology Club Podcast

- Dr. Paul C. Lin, MD, Private practice physician, Seattle Reproductive Medicine, 2018-2019, Incoming President of the Society for Assisted Reproductive Technology (SART), 2019-2020

- Kaitlyn Noble, Pre and post-natal health coach, personal trainer and certified Pilates instructor, Los Angeles

- Dr. Hemalee Patel, DO, FACS, Board Certified in Internal Medicine, certified in Ayurvedic medicine level 1 and 2, Lifestyle Medicine Expert, San Francisco

- Dr. Alison Peck, MD, FACOG, Physician at HRC Fertility, Los Angeles

- Dr. Meera Shah, MD, FACOG, Board certified Reproductive Endocrinologist and Infertility Specialist at Nova IVF, Mountain View

- Professor Amy Sparks, PhD, HCLD, Director, In Vitro Fertilization and Reproductive Testing Laboratory, department of Ob/GYN at the University of Iowa Health Care and President of the Society for Assisted Reproductive Technology (SART)

- Elizabeth Stanway-Mayers, RD, CSP, CN, Board Certified Clinical Dietitian, including pre and postnatal care, Lucile Packard Children's Hospital at Stanford

- Professor Lynn Marie Westphal, MD, Chief Medical Officer at Kindbody and Professor Emerita of Obstetrics & Gynecology and Director of the Fertility Preservation Program at Stanford University Medical Center

- Dr. Suzannah A. Williams, BSc Hons, PhD, Lead for Oxford Future Fertility Trust Cryopreservation Research Programme & Chair of Examiners MSc Clinical Embryology at Oxford University, England

- Dr. Ephia Yasmin, MBBS, MD, MRCOG, Consultant Gynaecologist and subspecialist in Reproductive Medicine and Surgery, Clinical lead of the Reproductive Medicine Unit at University College Hospital, England, Associate Editor of The Obstetrician and Gynaecologist (TOG) and chair of the British Fertility Society policy and practice committee

With additional advisory and expertise from:

- Amy Jewett, MPH, Assisted Reproductive Technology Team, Centers for Disease Control and Prevention

- Dr. Peter Klatsky, MD, MPH, double board certified in Obstetrics & Gynecology and Reproductive Endocrinology & Infertility, Director of Fertility Preservation, Spring Fertility, San Francisco, Founder of Mama Rescue

- Peggy Orlin, MFT, Marriage and Family Therapist Specializing in Infertility, Pacific Fertility Center, San Francisco

- Dr. David Sable MD, Former reproductive endocrinologist, Adjunct at Columbia University, Director healthcare and life science investing for the Special Situations Funds, Portfolio Manager of the Special Situations Life Sciences Fund

- Dr. Jenn Shulman, L.Ac., DAOM, FABORM, Jennifer Shulman Acupuncture, New York and Los Angeles

- Dr. Angela Tewari, Consultant Dermatologist, MBBS, BSc (Immunol), MRCP (Derm), PhD (UK), King's College Hospital, England

- Dr. Paul J. Turek MD, FACS, FRSM, Board Certified Urologist and Microsurgical Specialist, Founder Director of the Beverly Hills and San Francisco based Turek Clinic

- Dr. Juan García Velasco, MD, PhD. Director of IVI Madrid, IVI India, IVI GCC and Professor of Obstetrics and Gynaecology at Rey Juan Carlos University, Madrid, Spain

None of the expert panelists received or will receive financial remuneration or have any direct interests to declare regarding the contents of this book: their views are independent.

Disclaimer
While this book is based on information from doctors, the authors are not doctors themselves. The content provided is for reference purposes only and does not take the place of medical advice from your own physician. The book details the authors' opinions and interpretations of scientific studies about egg freezing. Every effort has been made to ensure that the content provided in this book is accurate and helpful for our readers at publishing time. However, this is not an exhaustive treatment of the subjects. No liability is assumed for losses or damages due to the information provided. You are responsible for your own choices, actions, and results. You should always consult your doctor for your specific health questions and needs. The term "woman" is used throughout this book for simplicity, but we recognize and respect that not every person with ovaries identifies as a woman. Every reasonable effort has been made to contact copyright holders of material reproduced in this book. If any have inadvertently been overlooked, the publishers would be glad to hear from them and make good in future editions any errors or omissions brought to their attention.

ELANZA Wellness can be found at www.elanzawellness.com

ISBN: 9781693410802

Table of contents

References
In an effort to not waste paper, you can find the references for this guide at
www.elanzawellness.com.

Foreword

As a physician and reproductive endocrinologist for almost 30 years, I can truly say that women have never had more options than they do now. For the first 20 years of my career, egg freezing wasn't on the table. If a woman was single in her mid-30s or 40s and knew she wanted to have children, she faced difficult choices such as being inseminated with donor sperm, doing IVF and freezing embryos with donor sperm or just hoping that someday soon she would meet her life partner and still be able to conceive. If it turned out that she was not able to conceive, donor eggs or adoption were the only options left. Today, assisted reproduction is no longer just about treating women or couples that cannot conceive, it is shifting to a proactive approach to family planning, especially if there is no partner in sight. This is of growing importance as both men and women are having children at later ages than ever before, despite their biological limitations.

The science behind egg freezing has been around for a long time - the first successful IVF cycle in the US occurred in 1982 and the first human pregnancy from frozen embryos was in 1983. The first birth from vitrified human oocytes was reported in 1999 and the field of reproductive medicine has never looked back.

Despite how far the science has come, egg freezing is still a highly technical medical and laboratory procedure and is still not guaranteed. In the lab, it requires experienced, trained personnel very familiar with in vitro fertilization and the exacting standards necessary not just to freeze eggs but to successfully thaw them and create viable embryos leading to healthy live births. That's why I prefer to refer to egg freezing as a "back up plan," even if many of my patients come in calling it their "insurance policy." Until the science advances to where we really know that 100% of a woman's frozen eggs can guarantee a woman a future child from those eggs, it is important to remain cautious and still try to conceive the way nature intended. Yet, the truth is that not all women are going to have that option. As we age, there is no reversing the reproductive clock. So, all things considered, the egg freezing process will allow some and hopefully most, although as yet not all, women to use this option to achieve a dream.

The decision about whether or not to undergo egg freezing is also a highly personal one for each woman. As with everything in medicine, patients must take the time to educate themselves about any medical process they undertake, especially if it is an elective and potentially life-altering process. I am very happy that, as well as containing the latest research and doctors' insights, this guide has been written by two women I admire who have themselves undergone egg freezing and have dedicated themselves to

ix

helping other women have better experiences. This guide will help other women gain a sense of empowerment throughout the process and I am impressed that the contents are based on sound, up-to-date medical evidence wherever possible, which can only help women produce better quality eggs.

That's why I think this book is a must-read for patients, doctors and other clinicians alike. If you do freeze your eggs, I wish you every success on the journey.

Carolyn Givens, M.D.
Double board-certified in Obstetrics and Gynecology and Reproductive Endocrinology and Infertility, Pacific Fertility Center, San Francisco, California

Note from the authors

Unlike periods, sex or menopause, egg freezing is not a universal female experience. It's not like you can just ask your mom or friends for advice. So, chances are you're feeling like 99.9% of women who set out on an egg freezing journey: on your back foot and on your own. Maybe you looked over your shoulder before you typed the term into a search engine, or you've avoided bringing it up in polite conversation - we've been there. The usual, prosaic line in blogs and magazines is that this is an empowering moment, so why does it sometimes feel like the exact opposite?

The truth is that most women we talk to are unclear of exactly what fertility preservation entails and how to best go about it. It's very hard to know where to actually begin, so picking up this guide and arming yourself with the facts and potential steps forward is a great way to start.

We know firsthand that egg freezing is not an easy process, but we also know that with the right information and support it really doesn't need to be so hard. Here's to being comfortable and confident in your choices, whatever path you choose.

Brittany & Catherine
Authors: Everything Egg Freezing and co-founders of women's fertility wellness company, ELANZA Wellness

Introduction: The "F" Word

Let's face it, the word "fertility" feels weird unless you're actively trying to have a baby. But, as with decent cosmeceuticals and eight hours of sleep, once you hit a certain age, fertility is just not something that can or should be avoided.

The word is laden with both obvious and hidden anxieties, insecurities, question marks and unknowns, and laced with political and economic pressures, as well as religious and cultural expectations. To the world, fertility acts as a barometer for the quality of your life, signaling everything from your health and vitality to your relationship status, financial stability, values and career goals. Fertility is such a heavy word that it can weigh you down, *but only if you let it.*

The first step in taking control is engaging honestly with the facts about fertility. This is not top of anyone's list but taking a proactive role as outlined in this guide can be a life-changing experience. It's never too early or too late to check out what's going on under the hood, get clued into the metrics, learn what options are on the table and what steps you could be taking to set yourself up for a smooth ride. Prevention is better than cure. Action is better than regret.

For much of our lives the care and advice offered to us about reproductive health is focused on one thing and one thing only: birth control. We're invited to forget we have a reproductive system or possess any working knowledge of it. Then, one day we're supposed to do a 180 and get pregnant at the drop of a hat.[1] The reality is that 12 out of 100 couples in the US have trouble getting pregnant.[2] Between 30 and 40 years old, not only does your chance of conceiving fall from 20% to nine percent a month, but at the same time the rate of miscarriage also rises from around one in six pregnancies at age 30 to one out of two by age 40.[3]

Suddenly, we discover that it's not actually always that easy to get pregnant and stay pregnant. This is a fact that is both highly personal and a compelling public health concern: overall, the fertility rate for the US has dipped below what's needed for the population to replace itself, which has big implications for sustaining things like the economy and the labor force.[4]

Thankfully, people are beginning to question the head-in-the-sand approach to fertility and transform what constitutes good reproductive healthcare, including preventative methods such as egg freezing. It's fantastic that you are joining that evolution towards awareness. This is your chance to step up and be one of the smart, brave ones willing to look the facts in the eye and give yourself more time and options to deal with whatever is to come. So, get comfortable with the "F" word and make it work for you, because from now on, we're all going to be hearing it a lot!

Why Doctors Say This Guide is a "Must-Read"

When you pay thousands of dollars for an egg freezing cycle, what you're buying is an increased chance to be able to have your own biological child someday. There's a lot at stake, and if you make the decision to do it or not do it, you want it to turn out to be the right one.

This book will shine some light on the biological, medical and personal issues you might be curious about at this juncture in your life. It will encourage clarity by helping you answer the question "should I?" And if that answer is yes, it will give you the practical tools and insights to go forward in the best possible way.

These insights are based on the best available research, the wisdom of over a more than 20 top fertility doctors and the personal experiences of dozens of fellow egg freezers. We wrote this guide in a way that reading it should feel like having all the best experts in one room, speaking to you directly and effectively at this specific point in your life, helping you come to the right decision more easily and helping you feel secure in your choices. You will find out: how the procedure works, what to expect day-by-day, what your outcome means for the future and, most crucially, the scientific evidence on the lifestyle modifications you can personally make that could help or harm your eggs.

It might not feel like it, but you *do* have some influence over your fertility. That is a fact now beyond debate. According to The American College of Obstetricians and Gynecologists (ACOG), your lifestyle choices can directly influence your fertility.[5] We spent more than a year analyzing over 3,000 studies from the world's most trusted medical and scientific journals and publications focused on fertility and the things that affect it to pinpoint exactly which lifestyle choices make a difference, and they're all contained in here. A healthy baby can only come from a high quality egg. So, you want to freeze the best quality eggs you possibly can, in case you ever need to go back and use them. And even if you decide not to freeze your eggs, these lifestyle changes you can make could have a positive impact on your ongoing fertility.

It's not too late to play an active role in your fertility, in fact, it's time to step up and take back some control!

How to Use This Guide

Everything Egg Freezing is organized into three parts, each containing information and perspectives chosen to be most relevant to you during the three different steps of your egg freezing journey. Although this guide is sequential and can be read cover-to-cover, you can also use the contents menu to skip to the most relevant sections for you, based on where you are in your egg freezing journey, or jump into particular topics you find most applicable. It's not a thriller, don't worry about spoilers!

PART ONE: *The First Step* - Exploring Egg Freezing

How egg freezing works, why other women are doing it, and the risks and chances of success explained. This section helps you start determining if egg freezing is right for you, even before you've set foot in a clinic. Reading up to the end of Chapter 3 will help provide context. When you're ready, use the latter part of this section to then figure out how to select the right fertility clinic.

PART TWO: *The Second Step* - Preparing Your Eggs for Freezing: Getting Fertility Fit™

Like all physiological processes, optimal fertility requires sound health. If you do decide to freeze your eggs, Part Two of this guide lays out a science-backed, 90-day action plan of lifestyle changes that you can start making straight away. The goal is to get your body and mind "Fertility Fit™" and into the best shape possible before freezing. Expect real, practical advice drawn from studies on what to eat, what to cut out, which supplements are worth the money and which lifestyle choices, changes, and tweaks are proven to help your body produce its best quality eggs.

PART THREE: *The Third Step* - Owning Your Procedure

This is your go-to guide and companion for all stages of the actual treatment and beyond. You can read it in advance as you're preparing, then refer back to it during the procedure and recovery for a quick refresher. It includes stories that help you figure out how you might feel physically and emotionally throughout treatment, ways you can setup good support systems (e.g. should you tell your boss?) and positive mindset routines that will help you maintain your cool no matter what the hormones throw at you.

PART ONE: EXPLORING EGG FREEZING

"Risk comes from not knowing what you're doing."

- Warren Buffett

Chapter 1: The Fundamentals of Freezing

"If you want the answer—ask the question."

— *Lori Myers*

What actually *is* egg freezing?

It's the fertility treatment made famous by Rihanna, Rita Ora, Sofia Vergara and a host of other celebrities. The New York Times reports that "lots of successful women are freezing their eggs," and Vogue deemed it part of a 2018 "wellness trend." It seems like everyone is talking about it, but what actually is egg freezing? Put simply: it's a clinical procedure to preserve some of your eggs. As you get older, your body will lose the ability to make healthy eggs, so freezing your younger eggs gives you an increased chance of being able to start a family at a later time.[6]

In an egg freezing cycle, you inject hormones that stimulate your ovaries. The resulting eggs are then retrieved, frozen, and stored. This is the same ovarian stimulation and egg collection process as for an IVF cycle, but your unfertilized eggs are frozen, instead of being mixed with sperm. If you encounter problems getting pregnant naturally in the future and need to have in vitro fertilization (IVF), thawing and using your younger eggs will increase your chances of having a healthy baby.[7] [8] [9] [10] [11]

Taking a step back, what are we actually talking about when we say preserving fertility? In essence, this means reducing the likelihood of you not being able to conceive your genetic child due to infertility. "Infertile" can refer to several things: 1) a disease where there's something wrong with your reproductive system; 2) problems getting pregnant or staying pregnant; 3) age-related issues, as a function of time where your body naturally ceases to be fertile, which happens to everyone eventually.

Egg 101
The egg is the largest cell in the human body, measuring around 0.1mm in diameter. Millions of eggs can be contained in the ovaries, which are around the size of almonds. An egg has a diameter roughly the thickness of a strand of hair, making it thirty times the size of a sperm cell. Unlike sperm, eggs do not have tails and therefore cannot move independently.

What do women who've frozen their eggs say about it?

"I found it was like a weight lifted off my shoulders. It's not like anything really changed and I get that there are no guarantees, but I'm so happy I got it done." - Kyra, 36

"The process wasn't that bad, it wasn't as big of a deal as people make it. I did it, I don't really overthink it now." - Stephanie, 33

"It helped me focus on what I really want out of life. I wasn't sure before if I wanted kids and freezing really gave me clarity on the fact that, yes, I do. If I don't meet the right guy in a few years I would do it alone." - Georgina, 37

"I don't regret it as such, but I met my boyfriend not long after I did it and I'm pregnant with my second child now. I could do with that ten grand back!" - Sophie, 38

"When I couldn't get pregnant and IVF with my fresh eggs didn't work, we tried using eggs I froze at 39. None of those worked either and it was devastating. I wasn't prepared for that at all and always viewed those eggs as my fail-safe option. I wish I had taken the facts relating to my age more seriously." - Jo, 43

"I met my now husband literally one week after freezing my eggs. I can't describe exactly what changed in my approach to dating, but I felt like I could truly be myself without being obsessive about finding 'the one.' For the first time, things just felt easy and natural and everything just fell into place. I hope this means I won't need to use my eggs, but I can't help but think that freezing them is what allowed it to happen in the first place!" - Charli, 34

"I feel in control of my life for the first time in a long time." - Joelle, 35

Why does egg freezing exist?

"A woman's peak reproductive years are between the late teens and late 20s. By age 30 years, fertility (the ability to get pregnant) starts to decline. This decline becomes more rapid once you reach your mid-30s. By age 45 years, fertility has declined so much that getting pregnant naturally is unlikely for most women." - The American College of Obstetricians and Gynecologists (ACOG)

As you get older, so do your eggs. There are a number of health and lifestyle factors that can influence fertility (as we'll discover) but, ultimately, the most important driver of declining fertility is age. As you can see from the chart below, while you might have a 20% chance of getting pregnant during your early 30s in any given month of trying, that dips down to around seven percent by the time you reach your mid 40s.

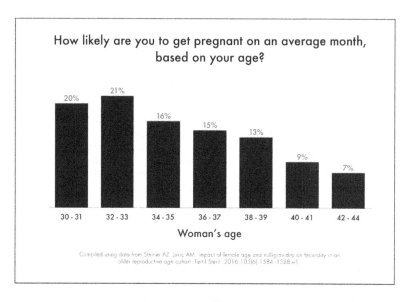

How likely are you to get pregnant on an average month, based on your age?

Woman's age

Compiled using data from Steiner AZ, Jukic AM. Impact of female age and nulligravidity on fecundity in an older reproductive age cohort. Fertil Steril. 2016;105(6):1584-1588.e1.

The reality is that infertility is an inevitable state for every single one of us around five years before we hit menopause (the average age of menopause is age 50-52).[12] The gradual decline into infertility can be accelerated by certain lifestyle factors and health issues, but - regrettably - no elixir to eliminate infertility altogether has yet been discovered. So, what's the best scientists have come up with to hedge against it so far? Enter: egg freezing.

Menopause

For most women, it is natural to experience reduced fertility at around 40 years old. At this point, you could start getting irregular periods as the start of the transition to menopause - a stage known as "perimenopause." This is a totally normal process and it can take up to ten years before your periods stop, usually around age 50 or a little older, though the range is anything from 30 up to around 60, at the extreme. When this process happens earlier or faster than normal, and periods stop before age 40, it's known as "premature menopause." This only happens in about one percent of women.

There is another similar sounding, but different, condition, that you might come across, which sometimes gets confused with premature menopause: primary ovarian insufficiency (POI). POI also affects around one in 100 women. This is a condition where a woman's ovaries stop working normally, but not entirely, before she is 40. It can even occur as early as during the teens. Women with POI have low levels of estrogen and high levels of follicle stimulating hormone, FSH, and menstrual irregularities.[13] The exact cause is often unknown, but POI can be caused by a disease, surgery, chemotherapy or radiation, genetic abnormalities, metabolic disorders, autoimmunity, infections, or environmental factors.[14] The difference between premature menopause (where menopause happens as usual, but earlier, and you can no longer get pregnant naturally) and POI, is that women with POI may still have occasional periods and might still be able to conceive, even where they have few functional follicles.[15] If you have menstrual irregularities that you're worried about, your doctor will be able to discuss them with you and run some tests. Menstrual irregularities are common, so it may be that they do not indicate POI at all and are nothing to be concerned about, but it's still worth discussing this with your doctor if you already have a family history of early ovarian failure, or an elevated follicle-stimulating hormone (FSH) level before age 40 years without a known cause, the ACOG guidelines suggest your doctor should offer you gene carrier testing, too, as POI can run in families.[16]

When is the best time to freeze?

There is no legal age cap to egg freezing in the US. However, as there is a lower likelihood of success the older you are, most clinics will only allow a woman to freeze her eggs up to age 45.[17] (That's presuming there has been thorough counseling on the low probability of success by that age.) Most doctors recommend ideally freezing before age 37, though, to maximize your chance of a good quality and quantity of eggs. That said, there are all kinds of factors that you'll want to consider. Don't worry, we'll discuss this in detail later in Part One.

Is it safe?

The top body overseeing fertility medicine in the US, the American Society of Reproductive Medicine (ASRM) says ovarian stimulation and retrieval is "well established and safe for women and babies,"[18] as does Europe's respected fertility body, the European Society for Human Reproduction and Technology (ESHRE).[19] That's not to say egg freezing, like any medical procedure, doesn't come with potential risks and side effects. We'll discuss those risks more thoroughly later in this chapter.

How much does it cost?

There's no sugar-coating the fact that egg freezing currently comes with a rather hefty price tag. The market has become more competitive in recent years as it becomes more mainstream, with newer clinics advertising services emphasizing relative affordability. However, the costs - in the US in particular - are still substantial. In the US, the average cost of one cycle is $12,500 (including medication) + storage ($500 a year), but the range is anywhere from $10,000 to $18,000 for one cycle, including medication.[20] You might see the most affordable quoted as more like $6,000, but that price doesn't include medication. Be careful to compare apples with apples.

Simplified cost estimate of one egg freezing cycle		
Item	**Cost**	**Notes**
Treatment	$6k - $18k	Includes monitoring, retrieval procedure, etc.
Medication	$4k - $6k	Varies based on how much medication is needed to stimulate the ovaries
Storage	$2k - $6k	Assume five years of storage, with the first year free
TOTAL PER CYCLE	**$12k - $30k**	

The range is broad partly due to the pricing approaches of different clinics, but also because there are a number of factors that influence the total cost of any one egg freezing cycle, with perhaps the most important being the amount of medication needed, which varies from woman to woman. Many of these variables are influenced by the age you decide to freeze your eggs (driving the amount of hormone medication needed), as well as the maximum age you would consider using them and the country you freeze your eggs in (storage costs over time.) Egg freezing is substantially cheaper in many other countries, such as Mexico (~$4,000), the UK (~$5,000), Spain (~$4,000), and South Africa (~$3,000). More on this in "Picking a Clinic."

Does it work?

"No one has figured out how to definitively extend fertility—yet. Egg freezing is the closest we've come." - MIT Technology Review.[21]

The egg freezing process itself does work. But that's not to say it does so every time, much like natural conception. In short, the medical technology can work, but it's not perfect and can't guarantee a perfect result. As things stand, you shouldn't *count* on an egg freezing cycle resulting in a baby.

The likelihood that one cycle will lead to healthy baby is still relatively modest and will be different for every woman. That's because a lot of different factors are at play, like age, general health and the quality and quantity of eggs frozen. For some women egg freezing might "work" in that it ultimately results in a healthy baby at a later date if she needs to use her eggs. For another, her eggs may not survive freezing and thawing, or they may not fertilize, or for many other reasons may not continue growing well. It is as fallible as nature.

As a rule of thumb, egg freezing has around the same likelihood of success as a cycle of IVF *at the same age:* similar to egg freezing, IVF is more likely to work the younger your eggs are. So let's say, if you froze eggs at 35 years old and then did an IVF cycle using those eggs at 40 years old, you will still have roughly the same likelihood of success as you would have at 35 years old, five years on. It's a bit more complicated than that in practice, but we'll get into the success rates in more detail later.

For now, what you need to know is, yes, the technology can work, but it's not guaranteed. As one of our Expert Panelists, Dr. Juan Garcia-Velasco, puts it: "women freeze their eggs, not their fertility." Frozen eggs might give you more of a chance at conception in the future, but that chance is just that, a chance, not a certainty. Your main focus should still be your underlying natural fertility.

"I froze sixteen eggs before I met my husband. We got pregnant naturally with our first little girl, but struggled to conceive after that. Our clinic thawed and fertilized my frozen eggs, which resulted in two embryos, and luckily from that we got pregnant with our second little one. We feel so grateful, especially with so many of our friends struggling to conceive." - Mariska, 42

"I froze my eggs when I was 38 and was really bummed when I only got five. My partner and I are going through IVF now and sadly, none of them fertilized. Now we're at the point where we're weighing up if we can afford one last shot with a fresh IVF cycle." - Paula, 44

How does egg freezing preserve your future fertility?

It's likely you will lose 90% of your eggs by age 30, and will only have about three percent left by the time you turn 40.[22] [23] The eggs that do remain are lower quality, which is partly why women become infertile an average of five to ten years before hitting menopause.[24] Egg freezing hits pause on some of those eggs. Your frozen eggs will remain at the same biological age at which you froze them.[25]

This is important because you're more likely to get pregnant using younger eggs. If you need to have IVF treatment in the future, using your younger, frozen eggs would theoretically give you a better chance of carrying a healthy baby to term, even with your older womb.[26] [27] [28] [29] [30] [31] Not only are you more likely to get pregnant, but you're less likely to miscarry and more likely to have a healthy child who does not have a condition such as Down syndrome or Turner syndrome.[32]

Scientists have shown that it's the age of the *egg* rather than the age of the womb than matters when it comes to getting pregnant and giving birth to a healthy baby by comparing fertility treatments where older women use younger eggs (from donors) to older women using their own older eggs.[33] Plot this on a graph and you can see that the women using younger eggs have dramatically improved chances of ending up with a baby:

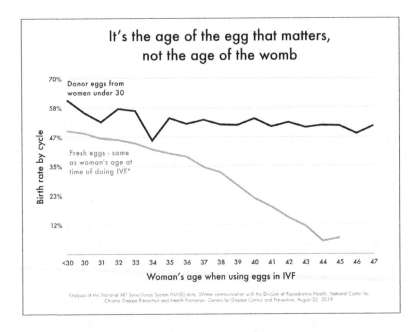

It's the age of the egg that matters, not the age of the womb

Donor eggs from women under 30

Fresh eggs - same as woman's age at time of doing IVF"

Birth rate by cycle

Woman's age when using eggs in IVF

Analyses of the National ART Surveillance System (NASS) data. Written communication with the Division of Reproductive Health, National Center for Chronic Disease Prevention and Health Promotion, Centers for Disease Control and Prevention, August 22, 2019

Although there isn't enough specific data yet to make a definitive statement, it's thought that if you freeze your eggs today, then use them later in an IVF cycle (essentially donating your current eggs to your older self), then you will have a similar chance of success as if you were trying to get pregnant today, despite your older womb at that time. The effects of aging on your womb aren't as pronounced as on your eggs. The point of this chart is simply to illustrate the difference in success rates using younger eggs, even when the womb is older - we'll discuss actual success rates later.

What does an egg freezing cycle involve?

STEP ONE Appointment with specialist (~90 - 120 days):

The first step is to get an appointment with either your gynecologist or a specialist fertility doctor - some women choose to go straight to a specialist fertility clinic, others get a recommendation/referral from their gyne. In order to understand if you are a good candidate for egg freezing, you will have to have certain tests run - these can be done either by the fertility doctor or in advance by your gyne (you can take the results along with you to the fertility clinic consultation so you can have a more informed initial conversation). The tests include hormones, some infectious diseases (required by most states in the US), and a baseline ultrasound. If you get the green light, your procedure can be scheduled.

STEP TWO Preparing your eggs for freezing (~90 - 120 days):

At this time, you can prepare your eggs for freezing by making fertility-friendly lifestyle choices that can optimize your fertility during the three months prior to treatment. This aligns with the window in which your eggs are rapidly maturing and will help your ovaries into the best shape for your egg freezing cycle. (See Part Two.)

STEP THREE Ovarian stimulation phase (~10-14 days):[34]

Once your treatment starts, each day, you'll give yourself an injection of fertility hormones, which are natural and modified versions of those normally produced in your body. In these higher doses, the hormones stimulate your ovaries to mature multiple eggs rather than the one egg matured during a typical menstrual cycle. Over the stimulation phase, you will need to go to the clinic anything from four to eight times for monitoring appointments. During these appointments, your doctor monitors how your ovaries are progressing through ultrasounds and bloodwork every one to four days and adjusts your medication dosage as needed. Some clinics may do additional blood work such as monitoring your estrogen levels. The actual day of your egg retrieval will be booked in the final few days of stimulation, depending on your progress, so flexibility with your work schedule around that time is crucial. When your doctor thinks the time is right, you'll take a final injection, referred to as the "trigger shot," which is injected exactly 35-36 hours before your retrieval surgery. This injection is meant to push your eggs to the final stages of maturation.

STEP FOUR Retrieval procedure (15-30 minutes):

For this step, you'll need to take a day or two off work. Despite the actual procedure only lasting around 15-30 minutes, you will need to stay at the clinic for at least a few hours for preparation and recovery. Your eggs are retrieved in a minimally invasive surgical procedure during which you will be highly unlikely to feel any pain. In most cases, you will be under intravenous sedation, which is milder than general anesthesia (no breathing tube needed), so you will feel "asleep" and be unaware of any discomfort. Then, your doctor uses a fine, ultrasound-guided transvaginal needle to collect the eggs from each of your ovaries. You should not have any outward facing cuts or scars. A lab scientist (i.e. embryologist) flash-freezes your eggs in liquid nitrogen into a glass-like state, to be stored in cryotanks until you decide to use them or no longer want to keep them frozen. You will be sleepy when you come around from the sedative and should not drive yourself home. You will probably feel like spending the rest of the day on the couch or in bed. Note that it is a regulation in some US states that a patient who undergoes anesthesia at a hospital or surgery center must be accompanied home by a responsible adult. Even if you live in a state or country where this isn't mandatory, it's still a very, very good idea to have a partner, family member or good friend primed to show up and take you home and ideally spend the day with you (the perfect time to binge watch that new series!). If that isn't possible, hiring a freelance carer or nurse (a trusted professional) to see you back to your home and settle you in would be a good option.

STEP FIVE: Recovery (1-4 days of discomfort & 10-12 days til back to normal)

You should anticipate up to three days of recovery. Most women are back at work the day after the surgery, but others report feeling significant discomfort up to four days after the retrieval. Doctors don't recommend any disruption or exposure to the vaginal area for 10-12 days after retrieval (that means no sex and no swimming). Nor do they recommend intense exercise that could potentially put your ovaries under strain. There should be no or only minimal bleeding - if you experience more than this, you should call your doctor immediately as something could be wrong. Your period should arrive after these 10-14 days and all should return back to normal.

EGG FREEZING SUMMARY GUIDE

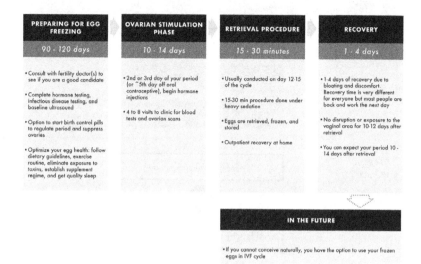

PREPARING FOR EGG FREEZING	OVARIAN STIMULATION PHASE	RETRIEVAL PROCEDURE	RECOVERY
90 - 120 days	10 - 14 days	15 - 30 minutes	1 - 4 days
• Consult with fertility doctor(s) to see if you are a good candidate	• 2nd or 3rd day of your period (or ~5th day off oral contraceptive), begin hormone injections	• Usually conducted on day 12-15 of the cycle	• 1-4 days of recovery due to bloating and discomfort. Recovery time is very different for everyone but most people are back and work the next day
• Complete hormone testing, infectious disease testing, and baseline ultrasound	• 4 to 8 visits to clinic for blood tests and ovarian scans	• 15-30 min procedure done under heavy sedation	
• Option to start birth control pills to regulate period and suppress ovaries		• Eggs are retrieved, frozen, and stored	• No disruption or exposure to the vaginal area for 10-12 days after retrieval
• Optimize your egg health: follow dietary guidelines, exercise routine, eliminate exposure to toxins, establish supplement regime, and get quality sleep		• Outpatient recovery at home	• You can expect your period 10 - 14 days after retrieval

IN THE FUTURE
• If you cannot conceive naturally, you have the option to use your frozen eggs in IVF cycle

STEP SIX: In the future

Usually, you will only use your frozen eggs if you try to conceive naturally without success. The advice is generally to talk to your gynecologist or a fertility specialist if you have frequent, unprotected sex but don't become pregnant after a year, if you're younger than 35 years old, or after six months if you're 35 or older. Then, after investigations and depending on the advice from your doctor, you might choose to use your frozen eggs in a process called in vitro fertilization (IVF). In this case, your eggs would be thawed and fertilized using either your partner's sperm or a donor's sperm (in a process called intracytoplasmic sperm injection, or ICSI.) Next, the fertilized egg (embryo) would be transferred into your womb. If it implants, then, bingo: you're pregnant. The same risks of miscarriage apply as for any pregnancy.

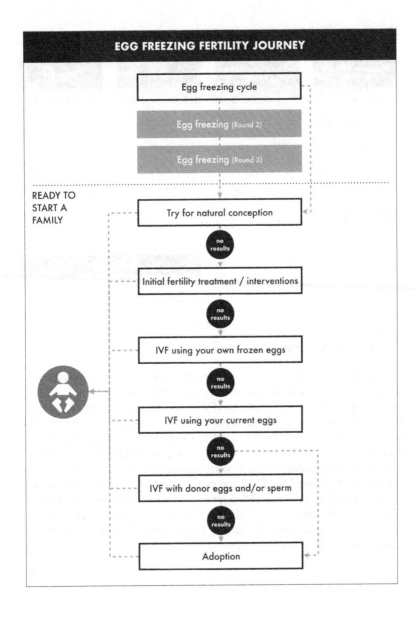

Will it be painful?

The injections can be intimidating but are generally painless

The ovarian stimulation phase is the part of the egg freezing cycle that requires your active participation: a daily dose of hormone injections. A member of staff at your clinic will give you a demonstration on how to inject yourself in your abdomen, right below your belly button. If they don't, make sure to ask. The needles range from about 1cm to 2cm in length and are very fine - similar to those that someone with diabetes uses every day. They're not painful, though some of the medications can sting a bit as they go under your skin. Your clinic will give you thorough instructions on how to administer these injections but if you have a needle phobia, you can always recruit a friend or partner and you can even hire a concierge style nurse to come right to you!

Injections usually commence on the second or third day of your menstrual cycle (depending on your doctor's advice) or after stopping birth control pills. The total time that you'll be injecting the hormones leading up to your procedure will be anywhere from 10 to 15 days, depending on how your body responds.

The procedure itself should be painless (due to receiving anesthesia) but you might experience discomfort during recovery

The procedure to retrieve your eggs is relatively non-invasive, conducted under sedation and takes around 15-30 minutes. A surgeon uses a very fine needle guided by ultrasound to reach the ovaries through the vaginal wall, bypassing the cervix and the uterus. There are no outward facing cuts, scars or stitches and you shouldn't feel a thing, though some women experience a small amount of bleeding, which is considered normal and should pass quickly.

Recovery, on the other hand, can vary greatly from woman-to-woman. From our own anecdotal evidence and that of doctors, it seems that the level of discomfort during recovery is correlated to the number of eggs retrieved. This makes sense if you consider the fact that each of your ovaries is about the size of an almond and that when you get to the retrieval stage of your cycle, you'll hopefully have a good number of mature follicles, which are larger at this stage, measuring between 1.2cm and 1.9cm each. As such, the more follicles you have (high ovarian reserve), the more your ovaries have to expand to accommodate them and the longer it might take for them to bounce back to normal. This is something to consider especially if you are egg freezing relatively young (and likely to have a high ovarian reserve) or have been diagnosed with Polycystic Ovary Syndrome, or PCOS. PCOS is characterized by overproduction of testosterone, as well as menstrual abnormalities. When ovulation does not occur, ovaries develop multiple small follicles. Because of this, women with PCOS are likely to retrieve more eggs and thus might need to tack on a few extra days for recovery.

DOCTOR INSIGHT: "Women with a high ovarian reserve often produce more eggs during their ovarian stimulation. While hyperstimulation can be minimized with certain types of protocols, the bloating and discomfort can still be more pronounced in these women, thus making their post-egg retrieval recovery more prolonged." - Dr. Meera Shah, Nova IVF, Mountain View

How many other people are doing it?

We're in the midst of some radical societal shifts: gender roles are being re-calibrated, both men and women are settling down later, and the concept of parenthood is being completely redefined. If you're feeling like an outlier because you haven't had a baby or settled down yet and people keep hinting at you to "get on with it," think on this: an estimated 20,000+ women in the US alone at some point this year will type the term into a search engine and end up at a fertility clinic freezing their eggs. It's also been a hot topic in the news, partly due to the controversy stirred up by major tech companies like Apple and Google, which now offer egg freezing as part of workplace health insurance. Even the US military is following suit.

It's easy to confuse the massive recent surge in egg freezing popularity over the last five years with thinking that it's just been invented. But, it's actually not a new procedure; in fact, the first human pregnancy from a frozen egg was reported as far back as 1986,[35] likely when you were just a baby, a kid, or not even born yet.

Freezing for fertility preservation reasons is growing fast year-on-year: in just eight years, there was a whopping 2,450% rise in fertility preservation cycles in the US, growing from 564 cycles in 2009 to more than 14,000 egg/embryo freezing cycles in 2017.[36] We asked the President of the Society for Assisted Reproductive Technology (SART), Professor Amy Sparks, what was behind the growing trend. She said, "The increase in egg freezing cycles for fertility preservation can be attributed to a number of factors, including increased awareness through popular press, direct to consumer advertising, inclusion of elective egg cryopreservation as a healthcare benefit and more insurance coverage for egg cryopreservation for women anticipating medical treatment that could render them infertile."

With these factors in mind, we predict that the number of cycles in the US will jump up to 56,000 by 2025.

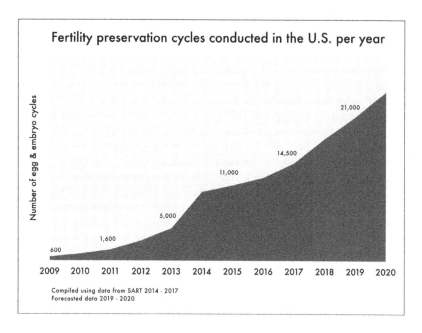

Egg freezing is now so mainstream that more than 99% of fertility clinics in the US offer the procedure.[37] It's also gaining in popularity around the world, including in developing countries. In cities such as Mumbai, egg freezing is becoming just as popular as it is in San Francisco.[38][39]

How did it get so popular?

We can trace the rise of egg freezing back to three key social, medical and technological factors:

First, there's a global "infertility epidemic"[40]

Maybe you feel like your fertility is a personal metric, but you should know to some extent we're all part of a worldwide fertility problem. The World Health Organization now identifies infertility as a "global public health issue."[41] Higher rates of infertility around the modern world are driven by two main factors: societal shifts towards delayed parenthood (in almost every country around the world men and women are having children later than they were ten or twenty years ago[42]) and also because many lifestyle factors, such as diet and environmental hazards, are curtailing our reproductive lifespans.

Think about it this way: the average life expectancy of an American woman has jumped from about 41 in 1900 to 81 in 2018 (a 95% jump), so it seems only natural to settle down later in life simply because there's so much more life to live.[43][44] The problem is that our stubborn biological clocks have stayed exactly the same. We know this because over the past hundred years there has been no significant increase in the age at which women experience menopause.[45][46] No, mother nature is not a feminist.

Teen pregnancy used to be considered a public health issue, but now, in the US, the teen birth rate is at a record low, dropping just below 19 births per 1,000 teen females for the first time since the government started collecting the data.[47] Meanwhile, have you noticed more and more friends having babies in their late 30s and into their 40s? That's not surprising. The most notable reproductive shift has been the number of babies born to women in their late 30s and 40s, which is the highest it's been since before the advent of modern contraception.[48] In many countries now, the majority of babies are born to women over 30 years old.[49][50]

Let's look at the 1970s for comparison. Back then, in the US the average age for an American woman to have her first baby was just 21 years old. That rose to 26 years old by 2016 and is likely to have risen since then. If 26 years old still sounds young to you, remember that the statistics include all women in the US, and the specifics depend on income, education and location, among other things. When you dig down into the data to just look at the women who live in big cities on the coasts and have college degrees, women are becoming moms for the first time far later than that. Living in San Francisco, for instance, the average age of educated first time mothers is 33.4 and if you live in New York City it's unlikely any lawyer or doctor entering motherhood will be younger than 33 years old.[51]

Researchers attribute the overall "older parents" trend to women having better access to contraception, higher levels of education and increased participation in the workplace, as well as the tendency for both genders to hit life milestones later than their parents' generations did: e.g. finishing education, leaving home and finding a life partner.[52]

So, why is all this leading to more women egg freezing? More people delaying parenthood means more people are experiencing fertility issues, or perhaps they are more aware that they could in the future.[53][54][55] Rising warnings and awareness mean that in turn, more women are being proactive about preserving their reproductive potential.

EXPERT INSIGHT: "I don't think the expansion in fertility treatment has even started. We have seven million women with difficulty conceiving but our most effective treatment, IVF, only benefits a little over 1% of them per year. Is there any other area in healthcare that is so underserved?" - Dr. David Sable, *Healthcare and Life Science Investor*

Second, regulators approved egg freezing for non-medical purposes

It's not just delayed parenthood and more awareness around infertility that has caused the egg freezing boom. Another reason it has become more common is simply that egg freezing is now an available, medically-endorsed option. Within the last decade, reproductive medicine bodies and regulators have publicly acknowledged egg freezing's safety and increased effectiveness, and have promoted it as a viable option, in light of increasingly alarming infertility rates.[56]

In 2013, the two main respected organizations of fertility doctors and other fertility professionals, the American Society for Reproductive Medicine (ASRM) and the Society for Assisted Reproductive Technology (SART), accepted egg freezing as a mainstream procedure and stopped considering it "experimental."[57] A big reason for lifting egg freezing's "experimental" classification was the publication of four randomized controlled trials (the gold standard in scientific evidence), which provided evidence that babies born from frozen eggs were no more likely to have genetic anomalies than those born from "fresh" eggs.[58][59][60][61] (However, we should point out that no long-term follow up of these children has been published.)

In 2018 there was a boom in media content about egg freezing, when it went from a Z-list procedure nobody had ever heard of to a superstar fertility treatment overnight: that's got a lot to do with the fact the ASRM released an ethics committee opinion that was more supportive about women egg freezing for non-medical reasons.[62] The statement effectively gave doctors the green light to talk to women about freezing their eggs for non-medical purposes, to preserve their future fertility. Or, as we now know it: planned egg freezing.

This is basically egg freezing to protect against your fertility declining as you age. Egg freezing was initially used for medical reasons only, for instance when a medical treatment was likely to compromise the normal functioning of a woman's ovaries (e.g. chemotherapy).[63][64][65] More recently, egg freezing has become popular with women who are healthy but not ready to start families, who are proactively planning for their fertility futures.[66][67][68][69] So, unless you're looking into egg freezing because you have a medical condition or you are going to receive treatment that could damage your fertility: this means you. You might also sometimes hear it referred to as *elective* egg freezing, or *social* egg freezing.

Third, the technology has improved, and so has the success

Retrieved eggs are now frozen using a flash-freezing process called vitrification. The invention of this process represented a great leap for the effectiveness of egg freezing. By freezing the eggs faster than the former slow-freezing techniques, fewer ice crystals form, meaning many more eggs survive the freezing and thawing process.[70][71][72][73][74][75] In 1999, you would have needed close to 100 frozen eggs to make one baby using the slow freeze technique,[76] but now it's around 15-30 eggs, depending on the age at which you freeze them.[77][78][79] (More on that later.) Biomedical technologists are constantly working on refining the techniques, so here's hoping the processes just keep getting better and better.

Chapter 2: Criticisms of Egg Freezing

Even a quick online search of the term "egg freezing" shows no shortage of strong opinions on the subject. The fact of the matter is, egg freezing is a hotly debated issue. This should not come as too much of a surprise given that the procedure touches on many personal issues including societal norms, religion, population dynamics, gender roles, medical ethics and, of course, an individual's health.

Before we [the authors] froze our eggs, we wanted to understand all sides of the story so we could make an informed decision for ourselves, not based on half-truths in news stories. So what are the criticisms leveled at egg freezing clinics, and, critically, is there any truth in them?

Does it give women a false sense of hope?

You don't have to look too far to find commentators accusing fertility clinics of "miss-selling" the procedure to "vulnerable" women as a way to boost their bottom line. Specifically, there is a suggestion that women aren't given sufficient information on the real risks and success rates of the procedure, leaving them with a false sense of security, or even a false sense of hope about their real chances of parenthood in the future.[80][81] While many women who have frozen their eggs say they're happy they did so, it's important to acknowledge that this isn't the case for every woman who has.

Those that are unhappy include some of the women who froze their eggs when the technology was less developed, and women who froze later in their thirties or into their forties and have returned to use the eggs only to find out that none of them were viable. There also may be some truth that the marketing of a minority of clinics give women a false sense of hope. Just as in any other field, there will always be variance in standard of care and ethics and a few people pushing glossy ads and saying all the things they think you want to hear.

However, the ASRM and its reporting arm, SART, issue minimum standards for practices to its members, including the guideline that doctors must properly counsel women on the risks and chances regarding egg freezing. Make sure your doctor fully explains your individual chances and risks based on your medical assessment.

Is it a fertility "insurance policy?"

Even more contentious is the statement that egg freezing is a fertility "insurance policy."[82] At a glance, it's an easy assumption to make: you pay money upfront hoping that you'll never need to make a claim but you can rest assured that if the worst happens (i.e. you cannot get pregnant naturally), you can "claim" back on those frozen eggs. However, unlike standard insurance policies, that payout may never materialize - in other words, your frozen eggs do not guarantee a baby. Knowing that, egg freezing is currently the only empirically validated means in which to reduce your risk of future infertility. There is no better policy being sold, so you could call egg freezing the best option available for some women.

DOCTOR PERSPECTIVE: "I tell my patients that they should consider egg freezing a "back-up" plan rather than "insurance" because there is nothing insured about egg freezing and women should still try to find a mate and try to conceive naturally, and use their eggs if it doesn't happen naturally." - Dr. Carolyn Givens, Pacific Fertility Center, San Francisco

Does it make women start having babies later?

The main question raised here is: if you've got your eggs on ice, does that mean you'll *purposefully* delay motherhood? The criticism is that women who otherwise would be having babies right now are delaying having them because they have frozen their eggs. Based on the research that says the main reason women freeze their eggs is because they haven't found a suitable partner or their partner is not ready to have kids (i.e. it's not the "right time" anyway), that seems unlikely, at least for the majority of women freezing. Understanding the real personal motivations of women who egg freeze rather than the media stereotypes helps to dissipate this criticism.

Does it distract from the need for more family-friendly policies?

Taking a step back to look at the larger ethical and social implications, some critics say assisted reproductive technologies (ART) like egg freezing fail to address the social aspects of delayed parenthood as they merely replace things that would mean women could more easily choose to start families earlier in life, like paid parental leave, affordable childcare and more family-friendly workplace policies. It's troubling, they say, because it's a medical solution to what is really a social problem.[83] In other words, if you subscribe to the assumption that women in their 20s and 30s delay motherhood specifically because it's too difficult to both be a mother and to have a career, egg freezing can be seen to function as a Band-Aid over what is actually a larger societal issue - insufficient family-friendly policies for both men and women.[84]

There's no doubt this societal problem exists. Women that do have kids when they're younger incur what economists call a "wage penalty."[85] A 2010 US study made this painfully clear, demonstrating how a year of delayed motherhood increased women's career earnings by nine percent and their work experience by six percent.[86] We love this passage from a research paper on fertility and public policy by renowned demographer Peter McDonald for how perfectly it encapsulates some of the deeply embedded incompatibilities between parenthood and a demanding career:

"There is...an insider-outsider labor market in which the insiders tend to be middle-aged males and the outsiders are women and younger people. The safest strategy for women and young people is to become 'insiders' and to delay or eschew family formation. ...In order to protect themselves from risk, individuals must maximize their utility to the market. This means that the need to focus upon the acquisition of saleable skills, work experience and a marketable reputation. At the same time, they need to accumulate savings or wealth as a personal safety net. They also need to maintain flexibility of time and place so that they can react to opportunities as these arise. The risk-averse individual in a world that rewards market production is unwise to devote time or money to social reproduction."[87] - Peter McDonald, University of Melbourne

Egg freezing has become a solution to this modern day riddle. Some say this isn't a fair solution at all, as it places the burden medically and financially on your individual shoulders, as a young woman and lets lawmakers somewhat off the hook from having to make changes.

The argument for more family-friendly workplaces is valid. But the question is, do individual women trying to find solutions *now*, within their reproductive years, really have to choose between the two? Why can't larger societal reform and an individual's egg freezing happen simultaneously? Just because some women are medically delaying motherhood, does that let politicians, lawmakers and companies off the hook when it comes to creating better, family-friendly policies? Suggesting women shouldn't egg freeze, but should instead wait for reform could be framed as asking a lot from young women in terms of personal sacrifice.

The truth is that nobody really knows how egg freezing will impact society and its existing structure. As yet, such a minority of reproductive age women have done it and are doing it that its impact is impossible to properly measure, but likely still minor. Let's also remember that freezing eggs is a way of helping preserve a chance of motherhood, not eliminating it. So those family-friendly policies are going to be important at some stage, whether that's sooner or later.

Does it make having a career and motherhood even more incompatible?

There has been some media backlash questioning the motivations of companies that offer egg freezing to their employees as part of benefits packages. Some suggest this "perk" is a tactic to encourage female employees to spend as much time as possible working through their reproductive years.[88] Of course, as we've discussed, women are waiting longer than ever to start a family. And, with a nine percent earnings boost for every year a woman delays having a baby, it's not surprising that HR managers report fertility benefits as being a top priority for female interviewees (also keep in mind that company fertility benefits cover both egg freezing and IVF treatments, making this applicable to both women trying to postpone motherhood and those actively trying to become mothers). But this also begs some larger questions: who benefits more from this, the employee or the company? And more contentiously, does this "perk" create an expectation that female employees will delay motherhood during their prime career-building years?

Of course, there is no singular answer to any of this - it's uncharted territory for everyone involved. But if you find yourself either a recipient or purveyor of these perks, there are some aspects of it that are worth thinking about. Employee fertility benefits can help attract and retain female talent. This is especially apparent in the typically male-dominated categories such as tech.[89] According to a 2017 report, fertility employee benefits such as egg freezing have been demonstrated to increase employee loyalty (61% of respondents) and commitment (53% of respondents).[90] So it clearly is beneficial to companies, but it seems far from certain whether that means in terms of forcing women to work harder or have children at more convenient times, or merely attracting and retaining the best talent. Additionally, some argue that encouraging employees to have children later in life could actually cost companies *more*, as the costs of maternity leave for older (usually more senior) women would be higher.[91] And the same companies offering egg freezing as a perk usually are also paving the way with more family-friendly policies, such as good parental leave entitlement, arguably making it a desirable thing to *start* families while working for them. The point is, egg freezing is a small piece of a big puzzle.

Takeaways

Fertility treatments aren't everyone's cup of tea. Sometimes folks are just plain ignorant and actually don't understand what egg freezing even is. That's pretty easy to deal with compared to other situations you might face - situations where people are actually fairly knowledgeable about what it entails, but they are suspicious of it or condemn it because of their belief systems, interpretations or fears. In an ideal world, everyone you tell that you're considering doing it will be supportive and open-minded. But the reality is some will clumsily orbit the topic with panic in their eyes then quickly move on, or, in a few cases, it might spark debate. In those instances, when we've faced challenges, questions or concerns from (usually well meaning) people about it, we've found it really helpful to avoid getting into a position where we're backed into defending our personal choice, but instead disconnect our personal decision from the bigger issues. Instead of justifying "why *I* want to freeze my eggs," the question can be turned around with another question: "do you think women my age really *want* to pay to freeze our eggs?" You can sidestep the question by opening up the discussion to egg freezing in its wider social and political context. Realistically, egg freezing is far from a perfect solution for everyone and it doesn't solve all the surrounding societal problems. Just because you're considering it or end up doing it doesn't automatically mean you have to become its biggest fan or defender! Absolutely, yes, there is a solid argument for wider policy change. And better regulation of the fertility industry might help reduce the chance that any woman would regret having the procedure. But ultimately, these are larger questions and responsibilities for politicians and medical authorities. In the meantime, for some women, egg freezing can extend their fertility timeline and increase their options in the future, right now. That's valuable. Whatever criticisms others may have.

EXPERT INSIGHT: "*I think shifting the conversation about parenthood choices, broadening fertility choices, advancements in technology, and social dynamics makes egg freezing the best option for women to extend their biological clock and allow for motherhood later in life. Personally, I am thankful to have access to the technology. Egg freezing is the most revolutionary advancement for women's health since the birth control pill in the 1960s. It has afforded women the chance to become older mothers using their own DNA, which is a beautiful future. It brings hope that women's biology can now catch up and be equal with men's reproductive abilities. Now, it is about understanding how the technology can best be utilized to assist women to extend their reproductive timelines.*" - *Valerie Landis, Fertility Patient Advocate*

Chapter 3: Five Facts About Your Fertility You Should Know Before Freezing

"A true teacher would never tell you what to do. But (s)he would give you the knowledge with which you could decide what would be best for you to do."

- Christopher Pike

1. You were born with all the eggs you'll ever have.

When you were born, you had around one to two million eggs.[92] So did your Mom, so yes, you truly are one in a million. Think of your ovaries as egg warehouses, rather than factories. They can't make new eggs; they just store them until needed.[93]

Did you know?
Your eggs actually existed before you were born, while you were still in your mother's womb. Because when your grandmother was pregnant with your mother, your mother already had all of her eggs, too. So your grandmother actually carried you in her womb - like some kind of cellular Russian doll. Baby girls in the womb also have around 6 times more eggs than they do when they are born - meaning the greatest egg loss actually happens even before birth![94]

---

2. Your chance of conceiving reduces with age

You've probably heard the alarming reports of fertility "dropping off a cliff" at 35 years old. But is that true? As we referred to it earlier, it's actually more of a gradual decline.

Between the ages of 30 and 33, there is actually no real difference in your chances of conceiving. Between 34-39 the likelihood gradually falls until, when you're over forty, you have less than half the chance of conceiving as a 30-year-old.[95]

In real terms, the best data we have indicates that in your 20s you have around a 25% chance of conceiving naturally each month, assuming you are generally healthy and have sex on a fertile day. In your early 30s, that reduces to about a 20% chance per month. After 35? You're looking at a 15% chance. Beyond 40, you can expect about a seven percent chance per month of actively trying. By the time you're over 45, your chances of getting pregnant during each menstrual cycle are considered less than 1% around which time you transition into menopause.[96] [97]

So, while fertility decline *is* more of a slope than a cliff, it's also important to be aware of the real likelihood you have of conceiving at a particular age and the unpalatable fact that, in simple terms, it's not actually that certain a process for most women to get pregnant, and it only gets trickier with each passing year. That's why it can take a number of months, maybe even a year or two, to conceive. And, even then, this only accounts for the ability to *get* pregnant, it doesn't mean that the pregnancy will lead to a healthy baby. Your odds of miscarriage increase with age as well. So, as you can see on the chart below, in your early 30's, you have about 20% chance of miscarriage but by the time you hit your early 40's, roughly half of pregnancies can end in miscarriage.

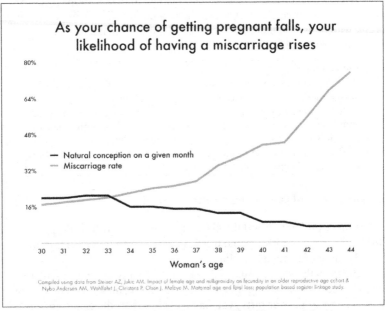

As your chance of getting pregnant falls, your likelihood of having a miscarriage rises

— Natural conception on a given month
--- Miscarriage rate

Woman's age

Compiled using data from Steiner AZ, Jokic AM. Impact of female age and nulligravidity on fecundity in an older reproductive age cohort & Nybo Andersen AM, Wohlfahrt J, Christens P, Olsen J, Melbye M. Maternal age and fetal loss; population based register linkage study.

Of course, this only tells half the story. The other crucial component is, of course, sperm. Here's a bit of food for thought: infertility is commonly billed as a women's health issue, but, in fact, 43% of infertility cases are also attributed to the male partner.[98] Men's fertility does also decline with age, just not as predictably or demonstrably as women's. Sperm freezing is rightfully getting more popular too!

3. Your egg count decreases with age

We're talking a lot about age, but let's dial things way back to when you were born. Back then you started out with millions of little pockets in your ovaries called "follicles." Follicles are fluid-filled, sac-like structures within your ovaries that house your eggs.[99] They're the kind of thing you'll hear about in fertility clinics, as they play a major role in egg maturation and the subsequent release of an egg in ovulation.[100] Eggs themselves are too small for doctors to see on scans, so egg count is actually measured by the number of maturing or "antral" follicles they can spot, also called the antral follicle count (AFC), which is usually complemented by hormone tests to give you a well-rounded view on what's called your "ovarian reserve." Your ovarian reserve shrinks over time as follicles are lost every month. So, even though you were born with one to two million follicles, this number will nosedive down to 400,000 by the time you hit age 18 and around 25,000 by age 37.[101] [102] When only around 1,000 follicles remain, menopause begins.[103]

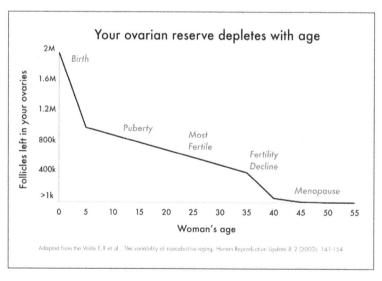

While the rate of follicle decline is slightly different for everyone (depending on a mix of genetic and lifestyle factors), age is considered the single best predictor of how many follicles should be left inside your ovaries.[104] What's important to realize is that while the number of eggs / follicles you have left in your ovaries is an important factor, it is not the *sole* indicator of your fertility potential: the quality of the remaining eggs also matters.[105]

4. The quality of your eggs decreases with age

A common misconception is that it becomes harder to get pregnant as you get older because you lose one egg per month and thus your eggs simply "run out." But as we learned, you started life with millions of eggs in your ovaries. So even if you are losing them at a rapid rate, you should still have a decent number left at, let's say, 35 years old. So, what actually makes it harder to get pregnant and stay pregnant with a healthy baby as you get older?

The answer is: lower quality eggs. A low quality egg, in simple terms, is one that is chromosomally abnormal. Declining egg quality is problematic for older women trying to conceive for two reasons: First, because a poor quality or chromosomally abnormal egg is less likely to make it through all the hurdles (fertilization, implantation, full term pregnancy) of getting pregnant and staying pregnant. Low quality eggs with chromosomal abnormalities are the most common cause of early miscarriage[106] - the older you are, the more likely your eggs are to be low quality, which is why miscarriage rates increase as you age.[107] Second, because the amount of DNA errors that occur increase as you age, the risk of your child having a genetic disorder, such as Down syndrome, rises abruptly in your mid-30s.[108] [109] By the time you hit your early forties, 80% of your eggs will be chromosomally abnormal, and that's what makes it harder to get pregnant and stay pregnant with a healthy baby.[110]

Your DNA by the numbers

Chromosomes are the parts of cells that carry genetic material from both the egg and the sperm. While an egg is maturing, chromosomes assemble in random order to come up with a unique combination, formulating the genetic "code" that creates half of you. Both the egg and the sperm have 8 million possible chromosome combinations. So if you multiply those together during fertilization, 8 million (egg) x 8 million (sperm) that = 64 trillion possible genetic combinations from a single egg and a single sperm[111] So don't let anyone tell you you're not a biological phenomenon.

So why are chromosomal abnormalities more likely to occur as you age? In short, because your ovaries are less equipped to conduct the highly error-prone process needed to mature a quality egg.

5. Your eggs take three months to "get ready" for ovulation

What was news to us is that your eggs aren't actually sitting in your ovaries fully mature. So that thing we said about ovaries being a "warehouse" not a "factory" is not *strictly* accurate. They're more like processing plants in that they make sure the crucial final steps to the finished product (a mature egg) take place. So, while your body can't make any *more* eggs, it is still constantly and actively putting important finishing touches to the ones that have been housed in your ovaries since before you were born.

Let's explain that in more detail. Over the course of any given month, hundreds of your follicles (the sacs that house your eggs) are called up to action (or "recruited" as doctors say). In an egg freezing cycle, the fertility drugs you take stimulate many more follicles to be recruited than in a typical month.[112] Up until then, your follicles have been dormant in a protected hibernation state inside your ovaries. Once recruited, they undergo a rather dramatic three-month growth and development sprint. This is all in preparation for their looming big moment: the chance to create the one egg that makes it to ovulation, and thus the chance to ultimately become a healthy baby.[113] [114] [115] The rest of the follicles that don't make it to ovulation essentially die off and get reabsorbed into your body at various stages of growth.[116] In a weird way then, your follicles are like wombs for your developing eggs, with ovulation being the moment of "birth."

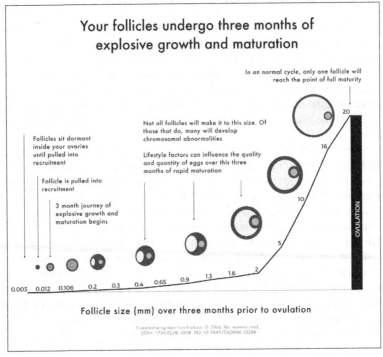

Your follicles undergo three months of explosive growth and maturation

In an normal cycle, only one follicle will reach the point of full maturity

Not all follicles will make it to this size. Of those that do, many will develop chromosomal abnormalities

Follicles sit dormant inside your ovaries until pulled into recruitment

Follicle is pulled into recruitment

3 month journey of explosive growth and maturation begins

Lifestyle factors can influence the quality and quantity of eggs over this three months of rapid maturation

OVULATION

20

16

10

5

2

0.003   0.012   0.106   0.2   0.3   0.4   0.65   0.9   1.3   1.6

Follicle size (mm) over three months prior to ovulation

Compiled using data from Erickson, G. Glob. libr. women's med.,
(ISSN: 1756-2228) 2008; DOI 10.3843/GLOWM.10289

What's incredible is that during their three "growth spurt" months, follicles can grow a huge amount, from 0.006mm (smaller than a grain of sand) up to 2cm (about the size of a peanut).[117] Remember, that's the follicle, not the egg itself. Here's what you should know: this window of rapid growth is an absolutely *critical* time when nearly all of the chromosomal processing occurs. If this takes place successfully within a follicle, you end up with a good quality egg, if it does not, for instance if there is an error in DNA copying, you will end up with a chromosomally abnormal egg. If a chromosomally abnormal egg is ovulated, it may result in the egg being unable to continue developing properly, not fertilizing, miscarriage or a baby with a genetic disease. So, what occurs in the follicle during the three months before ovulation is a central part of an egg going on to become a healthy baby.

BONUS FACT: Lifestyle factors can influence your eggs!

All this might seem kind of interesting but inevitable. Wait, we just got to the good part - what you can *do* to influence it. The science is clear that your lifestyle choices (environmental exposures[118] [119] and certain diets[120] [121]) can accelerate the ovarian aging process.[122] Your lifestyle choices could therefore impact the success of your egg freezing cycle.[123] [124] [125] [126] [127] [128] Are we trying to scare you into thinking that everything you've ever touched, breathed, eaten, drank, felt or done could have doomed your eggs? No, on the flipside, we're saying that the evidence therefore also suggests there are lifestyle changes that you can make that can potentially improve the health and functionality of your ovaries and, as a result, your eggs. That's because specific lifestyle factors are thought to play a role in determining and limiting reproductive years.[129] And that knowing exactly what you can do can hand a degree of control back to you.

Let's be clear, we're not talking about the fountain of youth here. Nobody has come up with the anti-aging silver bullet for eggs (yet). But with all this doom and gloom, we were excited by the prospect of even marginal gains, to make the most out of the expensive procedure. Even one more egg retrieved, or slightly better egg quality, could be the difference between your frozen eggs leading to a successful IVF procedure one day, after all. Not only that, but with the goal always being natural conception in the first place, ideally our natural fertility will remain so stellar, we'll all never need to use our frozen eggs in the first place. So, we dug into this and here's what we found:

Some well-known scientists claim that not only can you make specific lifestyle choices that can help protect your natural fertility in the long run, but that even in a relatively short period of time (the three months before your egg freezing cycle, let's say) then making some changes could potentially benefit both the quality and quantity of the eggs retrieved in your egg freezing cycle. That's because that "growth spurt" time is a potential window when the environment around your eggs really matters. Before the "growth spurt" period, when your eggs were suspended in a hibernation state, they are comparatively untouched by the destructive influences that other cells face - namely something called oxidative stress.[130] It is during the "growth spurt" period that your eggs start to come into contact with influences from their surrounding environment i.e. your ovaries. There have not yet been enough studies to demonstrate this to the point of scientific proof, but it is considered "interesting" and "plausible" by the independent experts in ovarian science that we spoke to. Despite the challenges with measuring the impact of these changes, plenty of doctors have their own stories to share.

DOCTOR INSIGHT: "I have a 37 year old patient that was diagnosed with premature menopause, deeming her completely infertile. She was no longer having her period, her hormone levels were completely out of whack and her hair had gone completely gray. I started her on a lifestyle program that included the tenants outlined in this guide and after just a little more than three months, the changes I saw were astonishing. Her FSH and LH hormone levels had returned back to normal levels for a woman her age, she got her period back and her hair color even returned!" - Dr. Hemalee Patel, Lifestyle Medicine Expert, San Francisco

So how can your lifestyle choices affect your egg freezing outcome? It all comes down to the condition of your ovaries and the lifestyle choices you make that can affect them.[131] While there is some irreversible damage to your ovaries that happens over time, especially if your ovaries are exposed to a very damaging environment (for instance, if you're a smoker - women who smoke even experience menopause one to two years earlier than non-smokers), by recreating the ovarian environment of a younger version of you - by establishing the best conditions possible - your ovaries are handed more of the proverbial "power tools" they need to create a higher number of higher quality eggs in the follicle workshops over that three month "growth spurt" period. Getting the conditions right can be like replacing a screwdriver with a power drill. And what are those lifestyle conditions? Optimized diet, the right supplements, how you're exercising, your everyday habits and patterns, from sleeping to what you wash with.

The exact details are all in Part Two, ready to help you get your follicles in the best shape for your egg freezing cycle, or at the very least, to know you've done everything you can to get the best outcome you can. Even if you decide not to freeze your eggs, the tips and tricks will make sure you're optimizing your chances of a healthy baby, naturally, in the future. What could be empowering than that?

DOCTOR INSIGHT: "Lifestyle has a tremendous impact on our health, so it also affects reproductive health." - Dr. Juan Garcia Velasco, IVI Madrid, IVI India, IVI GCC.

Chapter 4: Is Egg Freezing Right for Me?

"Knowledge you may get from books, but wisdom is trapped within you. Release it."

- Ismat Ahmed Shaikh

This is the big, fat question. The truth is, there's no easy or correct answer, and none of the doctors we've talked to believe there is a one-size-fits-all correct time or method when it comes to fertility planning. That's why it was very important to us to make this section really robust. It would have been great if someone without any agenda (either for or against) could have taken us through this series of questions to help us make our decisions and feel secure in them. But egg freezing isn't something a social media quiz can help you decide, and even a consultation with your doctor, which does cover the medical side of things, doesn't get right into the meat and bones of your own life choices.

Egg freezing is a deeply personal decision and not one of us has the same inputs into the decision-making process. Not to mention that there are some real downsides: the procedure can be expensive, it's uncomfortable, and there are no guarantees you'll even need to use your frozen eggs - let alone that it will even work if you do! But, on the other hand, egg freezing could be a good option for you right now, as it was for us: the procedure could give you clarity, confidence, hope and a sense of having done all you can to set up your future goals.

Whether or not you go ahead with the procedure, the questions that follow are an opportunity to sit with yourself and intentionally consider the bigger life questions that are probably lurking around the corner and one day might be banging on your door. It's our aim that after working your way through this section, you'll come away feeling more informed and confident in your individual choices, whatever path you choose to take.

EXPERT INSIGHT: *"Most of the women I talk to are either just learning about egg freezing and completely overwhelmed, or have been contemplating freezing for some time but feel frozen in making a decision. Most say they are scared of something small, like taking the hormones, when really their real concern is how much debt this will end up costing them. So understanding all the sides and decisions to make is key and critical to having a successful cycle." - Valerie Landis, Fertility Patient Advocate*

Start by asking yourself these key questions:

How do I really feel about being a mother one day?
Is it important for me to have a biological child of my own?
How many kids do I want?
What's my likely timeline?
Am I the right age to freeze my eggs?
What are the risks?
Can I afford it?
What's the likelihood that egg freezing will lead to a healthy baby?
Does it matter how old I am when I go back to use my eggs?
Should I freeze eggs or embryos?
Are there any special considerations I should factor in?
What had led me to explore egg freezing?
What are my other options if I don't decide to freeze?

Question 1: How do I really feel about being a mother one day?

Do you fall short of being a fully-fledged woman if you don't have children? Of course not. But, wow, does society expect it of us. While it once might have been unthinkable to feel no urge to step into the role of "mother," more women than ever before are doing so. While some women are childless by circumstance, for some it's by *choice*. It's something of a statistical trend in the West; one study suggests that almost one in ten women now make this choice.[132] Reasons vary from the more personal (no maternal instinct) to lofty (Swedish researchers claim that having a child is one of the most destructive things you can do to the planet).[133]

While people you know who are parents would probably call themselves "content" or "fulfilled," the data hints at a different version of the truth. An overview of studies actually suggests that "having children does not bring joy to our lives." It's counterintuitive, but for most of the parents studied, parenthood leads to no increase, sometimes even a decline, in satisfaction.

The research also points to a discrepancy between the expectations of joy that having kids will provide versus the reality. In essence, having kids might not provide you with the kind of happiness you anticipate having them will. So why doesn't having kids make us happier? Well, it's the same thing at play as when we think getting richer, or thinner, will make us happier. It's termed a "focusing illusion" - a cognitive bias we all get where we place too much importance on a single event. We think that event or outcome has the power to neutralize or override all the boring and bad bits of life (bills, worries, illness, arguments) but in reality, everything kind of stays the same. You get a bit more joy and a bit more trouble so, net net, what's changed? None of this is to say you shouldn't have kids, of course! It's just...having kids might not be the pot of gold at the end of the rainbow you might imagine.[134]

So, if you haven't already done so, now is the time to try on scenarios in your mind, talk to women on both sides of the coin and consciously consider whether or not you really *want* to one day take on the "mother" role for the rest of your life. It's a pretty big deal after all! And doing it for the right reasons (rather than purely because it's expected of you) is way more likely to lead to fulfillment and contentedness. To help get you started, here are comments on this from some of the women we've spoken to:

"I know I'm not ready for kids right now. I can't afford it. I don't have a boyfriend! But I know I want them and always have done." - Monica, 36

"I've just never felt maternal. But I don't know, maybe one day I will be and by that time will it be too late?"- Lana, 38

"I wanted kids, like, yesterday. But my boyfriend just isn't ready." - Cassie, 33

"Being a mother is not super important to me but I know my fiancé really wants to be a dad, so..." - Karen, 37

DOCTOR INSIGHT: "The most common thing my egg freezing patients come in and say is, 'I want kids, I'm just not ready now and I want to have more options for motherhood when I am.'" - Dr. Alison Peck, HRC Fertility, Los Angeles

ELANZA PERSPECTIVE: "Egg freezing made us both realize even more clearly that we do want kids, but that it has to be at the right time. Motherhood is a part of our life plans, it's just not the life plan – and that feels like a crucial difference." - Brittany & Catherine

Question 2: How important is it for me to have a biological child of my own?

Freezing your eggs, after all, could mean the difference between having a genetic link to your future baby or not, if you struggle to become pregnant or stay pregnant in years to come.[135] [136] [137] If this is important to you, you're not alone - 98% of fertility patients say they would prefer to have a genetic link to their child, rather than using donor eggs or adopting.[138]

We've established that using younger eggs (such as your own frozen eggs) could give you at least double the chance of a successful IVF cycle in your 30s leading to a baby. And if you end up doing IVF in your 40s, then using frozen eggs could mean as much as a tenfold increase in the chance of a baby.[139] If you don't freeze your eggs and you do become infertile and are unable to conceive using your fresh eggs, you might still be able to get pregnant, but that chance would be by using another woman's egg. The use of donor eggs (usually donated to older women by anonymous women under 30 years old, or a family member) has radically increased over the past decade, along with the rise in the age at which women are starting families.[140] Doctors tell us that when we see examples of celebrities conceiving in their mid to late forties or even fifties splashed around, the chances are good that they used donor eggs.

A surprising fact is that research suggests that fewer than 10% of people in the US and Europe who become parents through assisted reproductive procedures that used donated eggs or sperm, actually tell those children that they were conceived using donors.[141] [142] [143] The majority of kids who have so far been conceived using one or two donors, therefore, are unaware that their mother or father is not their genetic parent. Attitudes around this do seem to be changing with more parents starting to be open with their children about how they were conceived, and newer studies are finding that more like half of parents nowadays inform their kids of their genetic heritage.[144]

If you were to use donor eggs in the future, the latest research suggests positive outcomes for kids - with the caveat that there is a benefit to telling them about the nature of their conception before they start elementary school.[145] Those who find out they were conceived using donor eggs or sperm as a child or adolescent have a better response than those who find out later in life, or during adverse circumstances like a divorce.[146] [147] There's certainly far less stigma around donor eggs and sperm as it becomes more common, but some women prefer to freeze now and think of themselves as a potential egg donor to their future self, should they need one. Food for thought.

Question 3: How many kids do I want?

Except for the odd outlier like Octomom, most women or couples tell fertility doctors that they want to have two children, sometimes three. Isn't it true that we tend to only really think about the age we would ideally get pregnant with our first child, and assume if we manage to get over that hurdle...we should be fine to do it again? The reality is that some people face "secondary infertility," which is the inability to get pregnant or carry a baby to term even after having had no problem in a previous pregnancy.

Some studies even say this accounts for at least one in six (maybe up to one in three) infertility cases - pretty huge.[148] This is in part due to the statement that you're probably getting quite familiar with by now: people are starting families later. It's a hard thing to anticipate, but you should give extra special consideration to egg freezing if you're over thirty five years old and know you would ideally like several children. This doesn't mean you'd have to use your frozen eggs - ideally, you'll have them all without extra assistance - but you have the option should you need to use them.

Question 4: What's my likely timeline?

To help gauge this, you're going to need a pen and paper and do a simple thing we call the "fertility forecast." Everyone has a pang of anxiety around major life planning, but really, charting out life's scenarios doesn't set them in stone. The process just gives you a birds-eye-view similar to forecasting a budget or a business plan and can help you make the most informed decision.

Why? Because it's surprisingly easy for us all to think we have more time left on the biological clock than we actually do, especially when you factor in the small matter of, you know, actually meeting the love of your life, dating, living together, marriage (if that's important to you) and then the possibility that it could take a while to actually get pregnant. Or, if you decide to have a child without a partner, you might need some time to get financially prepared, and go through the process and practicalities of finding a sperm donor. If we had a dollar for every doctor we've spoken to who has a story about a forty year old woman waking up one day and having an "oh shit" moment, we'd...have a lot of dollars. This exercise isn't meant to depress you, it's meant to activate you – not into getting knocked up by the nearest guy (!), but into looking reality in the mirror and getting real with yourself about what it is you want and the path that's best for you to walk in order to get there.

Writing it all out in black and white is a first step in being quietly intentional with this area of your life and can help you get a better handle on the fertility realities of the age at which you might actually try for your first child, let alone when it comes to a second or third. Whether or not you decide to freeze your eggs in the end, fertility forecasting will help you realistically forecast the age you'll be when you might start trying to get pregnant and what fertility challenges this age represents. Trust us, don't skip this one. The simple things work. Give it a go.

The Fertility Forecast Exercise

- STEP ONE: Download the free Fertility Forecast template from the ELANZA Wellness website: ELANZAWellness.com

- STEP TWO: Put your current age in the top left column.

- STEP THREE: Now, in the column on the right, write out the potential steps to actually getting pregnant in the circumstances you'd be happy with. Think of it like this: if you're single, and even if you met the partner of your dreams *tomorrow*, realistically how long would it take before you would be in a place to think about starting a family, at the earliest? If you're in a relationship, what are the life events or circumstances that would need to come together for it to feel like the "right time?" Once you figure out the timing, match it up with your age at each one of those steps.

- STEP FOUR: Once you chart out the age you might want to have your first child (or more), match it up with the age-related stats on fertility that can be found on the ELANZA website.

Here's an example:

SAMPLE FERTILITY FORECAST WORKSHEET	
Age	**Life Event**
36	First date with "future partner"
37	Move in together
38	Start trying for a child
39	Have first child (if possible) **Age-related realities:** • There's a 13% chance of getting pregnant on a given month. • 25% of women at this age take at least 3 years of trying. • 38% of pregnancies will result in miscarriage. • 1 in 3 women over 35 require assisted fertility treatment.
42	Try for further pregnancies (if possible) **Age-related realities:** • There's a 7% chance of getting pregnant on a given month. • 55% of pregnancies will result in miscarriage. • 6% of IVF cycles using fresh eggs will result in a live birth. • By age 45, use of donor eggs is the only reasonable option for IVF treatment.

Age is just a number when it comes to most other things in life, but not fertility. Regardless of the lifestyle optimizations you can make to boost and preserve your fertility, for healthy women age is still the number one factor affecting the chance of getting pregnant and staying pregnant with a healthy baby.

Question 5: Am I the right age to freeze my eggs?

Statistics indicate that most women who freeze their eggs are between 36 and 38 years old.[149] [150] [151] [152] However, what's right for someone else might not be right for you. There is not one single answer to this question, as it must be weighed along with all the other factors like costs, your own life plan, and your doctor's advice. Here's what the experts say:

The best biological time to freeze your eggs is in your early 20s

That's when your egg quality and quantity are at their highest.[153] But increasingly the "prime reproductive years" don't correspond to women's readiness for motherhood.[154] [155] Plus, doctors rarely recommend that women freeze their eggs in their 20s because it is not clear by then whether it's likely life will go in such a way that they may need to use them.[156]

DOCTOR INSIGHT: "Many fertility doctors will discourage women to freeze their eggs in their early 20s because the chances of needing the eggs is so remote - they have time - and the technology may improve before their egg quality/quantity diminishes 10+ years later." - Dr. Eleni Greenwood Jaswa, University of California, San Francisco

The best financial time to freeze your eggs is age 37

When researchers from the University of North Carolina ran a cost-benefit analysis, it indicated that 37 is the age when women get the most "benefit" out of egg freezing.[157] Effectively, it was found that at age 37 women are "young enough" for their eggs to still be reasonably fertile, but "old enough" for the likelihood of using the eggs in the future to go up, making it more worth the price tag. Most experts agree that egg freezing is most successful for women younger than 38 years old.[158] In other words, women get the most bang for their buck at age 37.

That said, freezing your eggs past the age of 35 means you are less likely to get "good" results (both in the number of eggs retrieved and the quality of those eggs)[159] than women under 35 years old. In most cases, if you're over 35 years old you may require multiple stimulation cycles in order to increase the probability of a live birth in the future.[160]

Doctors recommend the best time is between ages 30 and 34

This is a balancing act with fertility on one hand and value-for-money on the other. Egg quality and quantity start reducing at around 30 years old. Freezing eggs at this time of life, when we have more sense of life plans, is more appropriate than in our 20s, as it becomes increasingly likely we might derive some practical use out of egg freezing.

ELANZA PERSPECTIVE: "We froze our eggs at age 32 (Catherine) and age 33 (Brittany) which is considered pretty early; we were some of the first of our friends to freeze our eggs, but neither of us feel like it was 'too early.' Practically speaking, we considered the fact that the sooner we froze, the higher the likelihood of it being a successful cycle and the higher chances of it being a successful IVF cycle if we needed to use our eggs in the future. From an emotional standpoint, we thought about how awful it would be for us and our (future) partners to cope with things like repeated miscarriages, an infertility diagnosis, and then having to endure multiple rounds of IVF, maybe even then without success – knowing we could have done something that could reduce the chance of having to endure all that."
- Brittany & Catherine

Question 6: What are the risks?

This is, understandably, one of the most common questions women have. We've laid out the general risks below, but before we get into them, we want to be super clear that this is a frank conversation you should have with your doctor. She or he can advise on a far more complete set of risks or expected side effects tailored specifically to you, based on your exact medical history and doctor-patient assessment.

The first thing to point out is that, despite the huge uptake in elective egg freezing, it's a relatively new procedure, so doctors and scientists are still building up the empirical data to understand the full risk profile. The data that does exist for egg freezing cycles tends to focus on non-healthy women, given the fact egg freezing only used to be done for medical reasons. This dataset is small - some figures suggest that only seven percent of women have so far "gone back" to use their eggs[161] - and, though it is informative, the data is not necessarily representative of healthy women undertaking egg freezing. As more and more healthy women go back to use their eggs that were frozen for age-related reasons, a more specific dataset will evolve. In the meantime, much of what is understood about the risks and safety of egg freezing is derived from studies that looked at IVF cycles. So, while over 2.4 million cycles of ovarian stimulation take place each year around the globe,[162] the ASRM cautions that there is not enough data now to know all the possible risks. The organization's guidelines state, "while short-term data appear reassuring, long-term data on developmental outcomes and safety data in diverse (older) populations are lacking."[163]

Before we get into more specific risks and side effects, let's cover some common, broader findings that address concerns you might have:

Egg freezing is regarded as safe

Despite their caveat about the size of the dataset, the ASRM says that "most of the medical procedures involved in planned egg freezing are well established; ovarian stimulation, oocyte [egg] retrieval, embryo culture, and embryo transfer are all regular components of IVF that are well tested, used worldwide, and regarded as safe."[164] The risks of egg freezing are similar to those associated with ovarian stimulation before IVF. If you have concerns, raise them with your doctor.

No causal link with cancer has been identified

This is a common fear based on reports that women receiving fertility treatment have higher rates of cancer (e.g. breast, endometrial, and ovarian), but in studies, no causal link has been identified. While some studies suggest an increased risk of cancer, most do not.[165 166 167 168 169 170 171] Researchers believe the correlation might be explained by surveillance bias[172] (women undergoing ART treatment undergo scans and ultrasounds which increases the chances that cancer will be found) or patient profiles (women who need fertility treatment are already more at-risk as a group).[173] [174 175] Studies have shown that even women with breast cancer are not more likely to have a recurrence if they undergo ovarian stimulation.[176]

DOCTOR INSIGHT: "In general, older studies linking increased cancer risk to fertility treatment suffered from methodological limitations – mainly failing to find an appropriate control, or control for confounders like infertility itself, which is linked with increased risk of cancer. The increased cancer risks noted were deemed due to differences in underlying risk factors in infertile patients compared to fertile patients, rather than the treatments. It is generally well accepted that there is not an increased risk of invasive breast, ovary or thyroid cancer related to fertility treatments. Long-term studies are ongoing." - Dr. Eleni Greenwood Jaswa, University of California, San Francisco

DOCTOR INSIGHT: "Hormonal therapy itself does not cause cancer. It can, however, stimulate the growth of cancerous cells. Therefore, if a person currently has cancer, or has a higher risk of developing cancer due to their unique genetic composition, hormonal therapy would be contraindicated. Before administering any hormonal therapy (for infertility or otherwise), doctors should screen their patients for any genetic abnormalities that may predispose the patient to cancer." - Dr. Aimee Eyvazzadeh, Private Practice Physician, San Ramon

DOCTOR INSIGHT: "If a woman is in any way concerned because of age or family history I suggest a baseline mammogram before starting stimulation." - Dr. Diana Chavkin, HRC Fertility, Los Angeles

DOCTOR INSIGHT: "Infertility is an independent risk factor for breast/uterine/ovarian cancer, however the treatments used [ovarian stimulation etc.] do not pose additional risk." - Dr. Meera Shah, Nova IVF, Mountain View

In essence, women who experience infertility are known to have higher rates of female cancers (which accounts for some of the scare stories), but these cancers are not caused by the fertility treatments. Research is still ongoing into the reasons for the link. Every one of the fertility doctors on our expert panel say there is no robust evidence that egg freezing will increase your risk of cancer, nor is there clear biological plausibility. The only risk may potentially be in women who already have breast cancer, because the hormones in an egg freezing cycle may stimulate it in a minor way, but this is still considered "irrelevant." Despite these reassurances, if you have concerns, especially if you have a family history of cancer, make sure to raise them with your own doctor.

Egg freezing does not reduce your risk of having a natural birth in the future

A common misconception is that by stimulating and freezing multiple eggs, you are "using up" eggs from your ovaries that could be used for a natural birth in the future. Don't worry, that's not the case. You would have lost those follicles and eggs regardless. In a normal month, your body loses around 1,000 follicles, of which only a single one usually matures to the point of ovulation.[177] You would also lose these eggs if you were taking birth control pills or during pregnancy. If it was actually the case that you have a certain number of eggs and you ovulate until they run out, stopping ovulation by taking birth control pills would then surely delay menopause!

46

(Unfortunately, that's not the case.) In an ovarian stimulation cycle for egg freezing, what happens is that a few of those other spare 999 follicles, which would normally be reabsorbed into the ovary (or "lost") that month, are stimulated into the next stage of maturation and retrieved by your doctor. You're effectively making use of some of the spare capacity. The fact of the matter is, you will only ovulate around 500 times in your lifetime out of all the millions of eggs you started with: 99% of the follicles are wasted.[178] There are plenty to spare for multiple cycles of egg freezing. In short, doing IVF or an egg freezing cycle does not lower your chances of fertility in the future, nor does it cause you to have menopause at an earlier age. This is because the eggs that are retrieved are eggs that would have been lost regardless.

Babies from frozen eggs are not more likely to have birth defects

About one in every 33 babies is born with a birth defect, also called congenital disorders. Not all birth defects can be prevented, though age is a big risk factor. Babies born via ART with frozen eggs show no more likelihood of having congenital anomalies than those born via ART treatments using fresh eggs.[179] [180] As such, there's not thought to be any difference in risk using fresh or frozen eggs. Even before the new, improved freezing technology came along, by 2009 more than 900 babies were born from frozen eggs and according to a committee from the ASRM, there was no apparent increase in congenital anomalies among these babies.[181] [182]

However, babies born via ART are seen to have more congenital anomalies when compared to naturally conceived children.[183] [184] [185] [186] [187] [188] Studies vary, but it's suggested that this amounts to slightly increased risk.[189] The thing is, this may be a case of correlation, not causation. Babies born to infertile couples also have higher rates of congenital anomalies whether they were conceived naturally or via ART, which is why some researchers say this indicates the treatment itself might not be the cause.[190]

So, if there's not necessarily a risk because of the actual technological process, why the slightly increased percentage of ART babies born with birth defects? Researchers make the point that women undergoing ART are already at higher risk of having babies with birth defects because of their riskier profiles: infertile women are more likely to be older, obese and to have chronic health conditions (like diabetes, high blood pressure, and epilepsy), all of which are independent risk factors for congenital anomalies in the first place.[191] [192] [193] [194] Women who have experienced a hard time getting pregnant or staying pregnant and who have turned to ART to help them have a baby may also have a higher threshold for abortion, given the challenges they have faced, possibly leading to more babies born with birth defects. ART pregnancies are also more closely monitored than general pregnancies, so more congenital anomalies may be identified simply because more are diagnosed and recorded. There are plenty of plausible explanations for the slightly increased risk that mean it's not actually to do with the process itself.

It's now generally agreed that there is no difference in likelihood of having a healthy baby whether a fresh egg or a frozen egg is used. However, we should point out that the fresh v. frozen studies done were primarily on women under the age of 35 years old - there haven't been similar ones on women older than that, so nobody can say for sure if there might be a difference after that age. With that said, studies are still ongoing into the link between ART and birth defects and more research is needed before the picture is crystal clear.[195]

Other pregnancy risks are probably not to do with the process itself

What is clear from the data is that women who undergo IVF are more likely to have twins, triplets and other riskier multiple pregnancies. However, that is usually as a result of doctors transferring more than one embryo into the womb, rather than because of the fertility treatment. It is generally considered now that single embryo transfer is best for the health of mother and baby. Ectopic pregnancy (when a fertilised egg implants itself outside of the womb, usually in one of the fallopian tubes) and the pregnancy complication preeclampsia (with symptoms including high blood pressure) appear to be more common in assisted conception than in natural conception. However, researchers think that the increased risk of these conditions is most likely related to a woman's fertility problems and the fact she's more likely to be carrying more than one baby at a time."[196] As a result, it's not thought to be the actual processes of assisted conception increases these risks.

You can expect some short-term side effects

The short-term side effects of the procedure are clear and are generally minor. (Long term side effects are considered safe, but, as with all things in egg freezing, are still being studied.)

While there are usually no dramatic or serious side effects, the main thing you should expect is that during and immediately after ovulation stimulation and egg retrieval, your ovaries will be enlarged due to the stimulation hormones, which can feel really uncomfortable. For most women, this temporary bloating and some PMS-like symptoms are the extent of the egg freezing side effects. These side effects should only last for the days the medication is taken and subside a few days after the procedure. There are some other things to watch out for though:

Likely:

- **Bloating** - During stimulation and for several days after retrieval, a degree of abdominal bloating is common and expected.

- **PMS-like symptoms** - This might include headaches, mood swings, insomnia, hot or cold flashes, breast tenderness, mild fluid retention.

- **Fatigue** - This isn't just when recovering from the sedative after retrieval, but can manifest during the hormone injection period, too. Think of it a bit like how your energy levels can fluctuate during your menstrual cycle along with hormones.

- **Bruising** - The hormone injection site on your abdomen could become sore, red, or slightly bruised. Switching up the injection site throughout the process can help with that.

- **Grogginess after retrieval** - The sedative used for the retrieval procedure is similar to that used by dentists for wisdom tooth extractions. It's commonly a propofol-based sedation medication sometimes called "twilight" anesthesia or a "deep sleep" and is monitored anesthesia care. It carries an extremely low risk of complications and doesn't require a breathing tube. Still, you'll probably feel groggy afterward as it wears off (like a sleeping pill), which is why you won't be able to drive home.

Somewhat likely:

- **Cramping** - After the retrieval procedure, some women report feeling discomfort around the ovaries and lower abdomen due to puncture sites on the ovary and the vagina.

Rare:

- **Menstrual cycle problems** - Your menstrual cycle should return to normal with a period one to two weeks following the procedure, though some women do experience spotting. Speak to your doctor if you do not get a period within two weeks of the procedure. The next period is sometimes delayed as the body "resets."

Very rare:

- **Bleeding or infection** - Bleeding as a result of the procedure can happen, but this is extremely rare. If you experience symptoms like the ones below call your clinic. According to Dr. Eleni Greenwood Jaswa, "Bleeding after a procedure may accumulate in the belly and cause abdominal/pelvic pain, shoulder pain (the nerves irritated by blood in the abdomen are sensed in the shoulder), dizziness, lightheadedness, feeling faint or weak. Often, women who have procedural bleeding into their belly will not be seeing vaginal bleeding."

  - **Infection** - Infection as a result of the procedure can also happen, but this is also extremely rare. Some clinics may give antibiotics to prevent infections.

- **Moderate Ovarian Hyperstimulation Syndrome (OHSS)** – This affects less than five percent of women. Mild-to-moderate ovarian hyperstimulation syndrome involves fatigue, nausea, headaches, abdominal pain, breast tenderness, and irritability, but these adverse effects can usually be well-controlled.[197]

  - **Severe Ovarian Hyperstimulation Syndrome (OHSS)** – This affects less than one percent of women. (NOTE: Many clinics have been replacing the use of hCg as the trigger shot with GnRHa instead, which advocates of that treatment protocol say has greatly decreased OHSS in the last five years, especially for at-risk women.)[198] Symptoms of moderate OHSS include extreme bloating, thirst and dehydration. You may only pass small amounts of urine, which are dark in color, and/or you may experience difficulty breathing, abdominal pain, dehydration, and vomiting. A serious, but rare, complication is the formation of a blood clot (thrombosis) in the legs or lungs. The symptoms of this are a swollen, tender leg or pain in your chest and breathlessness.[199] A very small number of deaths due to OHSS have been reported. Although there is no treatment that can reverse OHSS, it will usually get better with time.[200] Severe OHSS can be thought of as the loss of control over stimulation of the ovaries.[201] With careful dosing and monitoring, most cases can be avoided. If you have concerns about OHSS, raise these with your doctor. Note that the risk is higher if you are under 30 years old (as you are more likely to have a higher number of eggs),[202] if you've had OHSS before, if you have PCOS,[203] [204] or if you have other medical problems like hypertension, diabetes, obesity, hypothyroidism or anemia.[205]

- **Anesthesia risk** - Less than one percent risk of difficulty breathing and low blood oxygen for women of normal weight, but of more concern for obese women.[206] Where general anesthesia is used, it comes with its own set of risks, which is proportionately higher for women that are obese. This is why many clinics have upper limits for BMI for the patients they will treat. Make sure to let your doctor or nurse know if you have ever had a reaction to an anesthetic or sedative, or if you are allergic to any medications.

- **Damage to nearby organs like bowel/bladder/blood vessels** - Less than one percent risk. The procedure is performed under transvaginal ultrasound guidance to avoid this complication.[207]

  - **Ovarian torsion** - Though very rare, an ovary may twist around the ligaments that hold it in place, potentially cutting off blood flow to the ovary and fallopian tube.[208] The chance is slightly increased due to their enlargement. To avoid ovarian torsion, many clinics recommend avoiding vigorous exercise during and after the treatment cycle until the ovaries have returned to their normal size.[209]

- **Pregnancy** - Although rare, this can happen. A lot of clinics recommend not having sex during an egg freezing cycle.

Your own medical history and individual health may mean an increased risk of one or more of these side effects, so always discuss these with your doctor at length.

"I felt fine most of the time. I just felt a bit tired." - Shannon, 36

"I found the bloating really, really uncomfortable. I couldn't sit still and things didn't properly go back to normal until about a week after my procedure." - Hannah, 33

DOCTOR INSIGHT: "Feeling fatigued is probably the most common complaint/feedback I get during stimulation and is not necessarily due to OHSS. I tell my patients, when counseling them on how they may feel, is that in almost 30 years of doing this, I cannot remember a single patient who stopped her medications prior to egg retrieval due to side effects." - Dr. Diana Chavkin, HRC Fertility, Los Angeles

Question 7: Can I afford it?

Egg freezing is a spendy procedure. Especially for something that doesn't come with a 100% guarantee. With average costs of around $12,500 (plus storage fees of around $500 per year), it's not within reach for everyone. Unless money is no object, how can you figure out if it's going to be something you can realistically do? Relevant inputs to understand the total cost include the location you want to freeze your eggs, your current age, how many cycles you might need, and what your financing options are.

Before we look at some of the practicalities, let's take a moment to step back to put cost in a larger perspective and think about whether egg freezing should even be framed as a spend, as it often is, or more of an investment.

Could egg freezing actually represent a saving?

Egg freezing is a big expense, yes, but when you put the price into perspective, it might start feeling like a better deal. Researchers have estimated that egg freezing at, say, age 35 and using the eggs at age 40, could potentially save you $15,000, rather than waiting until you're 40 and trying to become pregnant and needing fertility treatment at that time. It makes sense if you consider that once you turn 40, there's only a nine percent chance that you'll conceive naturally in one menstrual cycle[210] and IVF treatments at age 40 give you only slightly more chance at 15% per cycle. The reason IVF success rates are so low at that age is because you would be using your "fresh eggs," or rather, the eggs that match your age versus using younger, frozen eggs. For example, if you froze when you were 35 and used those eggs in IVF at age 40, your chance of success jumps up to 26%.[211]

The lower success rates using fresh eggs translates to higher costs because you'd probably need to undergo multiple cycles.[212] In the US the price of one cycle of IVF will run you about $23k and most women will need around two to three cycles. This nets out to about $50k to have a baby.[213] And then, if after multiple cycles you still can't conceive, you might choose to get donor eggs from another, younger woman. The cost to do this can be around $40k. On the other hand, if you freeze your own eggs, you essentially function as your own egg donor, which means that off the bat, you've got a better chance of being successful. Of course, you might end up not using your frozen eggs at all. Nobody has a crystal ball, unfortunately, so the savings are theoretical. It's definitely a different way to think about it, though.

What's the relative value to me?

Some things are really valuable in the long-term and some things are kind of...not. The point is that context is king when it comes to assigning a large sum of money to something. When you think of egg freezing in terms of piece of mind and long-term quality of life investment, it starts to feel more like an investment in something like your education or 401K than something like a handbag or a vacation, right? That's why it's probably right to consider egg freezing costs in the context of your whole life, not just your life right now. It's essential to be responsible and consider how it fits into your wider financial picture, absolutely, but, in the end, what you assign your money to is a factor of what is truly important to you in the long run.

On average, women do two cycles of egg freezing

Something else that factors into affordability is how many cycles you're likely to need to make egg freezing worthwhile. As we've discussed, the more eggs you freeze, the higher the likelihood that those eggs could lead to a baby in the future. Comparatively older women are far more likely to choose to do multiple cycles, sometimes even four or five, which can bring up the average.

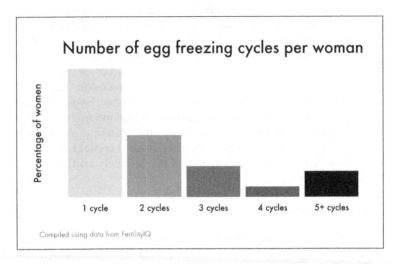

Number of egg freezing cycles per woman

Compiled using data from FertilityIQ

A 30 year old might retrieve 15 eggs from one cycle and, given the quality is likely to be good at that age, she may be satisfied with stopping there. On the other hand, a 38 year old woman might retrieve six eggs from one cycle and decide to do a further cycle or two to freeze a total number she is more satisfied with.

If you are advised to consider two or three cycles, or you would like to, bear in mind that you won't necessarily calculate the cost of these cycles by multiplying the cost of a single cycle by two or three. An abundance of clinics have multi-cycle deals, which can make the cost-per-cycle more manageable. Some women, particularly those with lower ovarian reserves, even opt for "egg quantity" deals, where you pay a flat rate for a minimum number of eggs to be retrieved, rather than paying out per cycle.

DOCTOR PERSPECTIVE: "One important consideration is that if you are going to use your eggs at a time when you're getting close to menopause, then you should plan on freezing more eggs. I have seen too many women freeze eggs when they're 32 and come back at age 42 - a time when they're menopausal - to find out that their eggs didn't work and now they're out of options." - Dr. Aimee Eyvazzadeh, Private Practice Physician, San Ramon

Does health insurance cover egg freezing?

The increasingly prominent debate on whether public policy around child care should better enable women to have children when their fertility is at its best also extends to questions of finance.[214] But while pregnancy coverage was introduced as an essential health benefit in the Affordable Care Act (ACA), unfortunately, planned egg freezing or even other fertility treatments are not covered.[215] (Surprising, given infertility is classified as a "disease of the reproductive system" by the World Health Organization.[216]) In part, the exclusion is because planned egg freezing is currently considered "elective" surgery.

That's a viewpoint that is increasingly being challenged, including by David Sable, a former fertility doctor and now healthcare investor and Columbia University adjunct professor, who questions why we don't label egg freezing as preventative healthcare.

Until the semantics and perception of egg freezing shift to being a form of preventative care rather than elective procedure, it's tough to make headway in the insurance conundrum. A small help, however, is that currently some insurance plans might cover the cost of some or all of the diagnostic tests ($175-$700), as well as the initial fertility consultation fee ($200-$300). Company and individual plans can offer more extensive fertility coverage, but it's not required. That said a growing number of companies like Pinterest, Spotify, Unilever, Chanel, Bank of America, Bain and even the City of Baltimore government have led the way by offering fertility treatment as a benefit to their employees.[217]

Perhaps your company doesn't offer this now but some of the women we've spoken to have been able to have it added to their standard insurance.

"I had heard of other companies offering it as a benefit so I thought, 'It doesn't hurt to ask. The worst thing they can say is no.' So I spoke to HR. They took it on board and amazingly it's part of our employee insurance policy now! Turns out it was on their radar already, and a few colleagues had already asked about it too. I'm so happy I spoke up." - Becca, 36

Are there alternative financing options?

- **Subscription plans** - Third party lenders offer some egg freezing financing options that allow you to make monthly payments instead of paying for it all in one go.[218] Treat this like any financial decision - do your homework, seek plenty of expert advice, select a reputable firm and be cautious about entering into debt. However monthly payments are sold to you, it's still essentially debt.

- **Freeze-now-pay-later** - Some clinics now offer built-in financing options directly.

- **Family support** - There are reports of parents chipping in to help their adult daughters preserve fertility - in essence buying their own insurance policy to have grandkids one day. One prominent British fertility doctor even says she thinks it will become "the new 30th birthday present." [219]

- **Crowdfunding** - There is a rise in women crowdfunding their fertility treatments on platforms like Kickstarter, Indigogo or iFundWomen. While not for everyone, maybe this is the next wave in fertility trends!

Is it cheaper to freeze my eggs overseas?

Medical costs in the US are substantially more than in other countries in general, and egg freezing costs around three or four times the global average! No surprise then that, as the world is getting smaller and we're all traveling more, fertility tourism is gaining in popularity. But how popular is popular? Globally, it's estimated that nearly a million people a year go overseas for reproductive health care like fertility treatments - so quite a lot! Some prestigious US medical centers, including Harvard, Boston University, Johns Hopkins, and the Cleveland Clinic, have even established hospitals and clinics outside of the United States, possibly to capitalize on medical tourism.[220] [221] That being said, despite the growing numbers, still only a tiny percentage of overall fertility patients leave the US for treatment.[222]

The main motivation is price point. Many safe and medically reputable countries offer procedures at 30%-65% the cost of care in the United States.[223] Lower overheads, staff salary costs and lower malpractice insurance costs make this possible.[224] Countries known for fertility tourism include Spain, Mexico, India and now even less obvious destinations such as the Cayman Islands.

"Freezing my eggs overseas required additional research and logistics. I had my doubts while I was planning. But I established a relationship with the doctor via email and video call before I traveled, which increased my confidence. Fortunately, the entire process was smooth. The doctor and nurses were caring and thorough and professional. I ended up spending a fraction of what it would've cost in NYC, and I got a relaxing beach vacation out of it!" - Sharman, 33

ELANZA PERSPECTIVE: "We both froze our eggs in Cape Town, South Africa, which is known as a medical tourism destination with some great state-of-the-art clinics. It was dramatically more affordable than in the US (around a quarter of the price) and the UK (around half the price). While having treatment overseas isn't for everyone, it really worked for our circumstances." - Brittany & Catherine

DOCTOR INSIGHT: "We see a lot of women from countries where egg freezing is not allowed (like Israel, or, until recently, the UAE) or from countries where they do not have as much experience. The good thing is that the women can do all the monitoring locally with their doctors and only need to come for 1 day for the retrieval. Sometimes they come just because it is significantly cheaper than in their countries." - Dr. Juan García Velasco, IVI Madrid, IVI India, IVI GCC

EXPERT INSIGHT: "Freezing your eggs is often an emotional and logistically challenging experience, especially if you're juggling work, hiding symptoms from colleagues, and going to really early appointments, not to mention the financial burden placed on patients with treatment costs of up to $20k in the US. Women have told us that doing the procedure on vacation abroad, sometimes even together with other friends, turns it into a much more empowering and relaxed experience. By going abroad, women can also benefit from more affordable treatments at top clinics, where salaries are lower, competition is higher, and drug prices are more regulated. It's critical to vet fertility clinics to make sure you're not compromising on quality of care and outcomes." - Kathy Gerlach, CEO Ovally (a company that arranges fertility treatment vacations in Spain).

The reverse of American women traveling to other countries, the US is a big fertility tourism destination in its own right. Much of this can be attributed to the less restrictive laws around ART.

DOCTOR INSIGHT: "We have many women from other countries come to our clinic to freeze eggs and do IVF. If they are with us for the entire egg retrieval process it takes about 2 weeks. Very rarely will they need to be in the US longer than that. And many women choose to do their monitoring overseas at home and then come in a few days before their retrieval. We have women fly home the next day and don't see a reason to keep them in the US for several days." - Dr. Diana Chavkin, HRC Fertility, Los Angeles

Question 8: What is the likelihood that egg freezing will lead to a healthy baby?

Ah, if only this question was just that simple to answer. In general, the chance of achieving a successful pregnancy using IVF treatment (which is how you would use your frozen eggs) is about 2%-35% for each cycle, depending on the age of the eggs used. This doesn't sound that great, but to put it in perspective, the chance of success in ART treatments is roughly six percent higher than your odds of conceiving without assistance on a given month.[225] [226]

However, some clinicians on our Expert Panel actually quote IVF success rates of up to 50% per cycle. This is most often the case when the eggs are younger, there are more eggs retrieved during the cycle, and when preimplantation genetic testing is conducted on embryos prior to implantation. Because freezing, thawing and IVF are not fail-safe processes, some doctors recommend doing multiple egg freezing cycles to bank as many eggs as possible.

But we're still dealing with "known unknowns." The truth is that even after your eggs are retrieved (i.e. once you know how many mature eggs are suitable enough to be frozen), you won't know for sure if any one of these eggs will be capable of becoming a healthy baby one day. One reason for this is that there is to date no technology that can accurately measure the quality of your eggs (although some technologies currently in development might make this possible in the near future). In lieu of this, embryologists follow specific guidelines to determine which eggs are most mature. The logic being that mature eggs are more likely to have gone through all the phases of chromosomal processing in order to be deemed good quality. Despite this, as it currently stands, only eggs that have been successfully fertilized by sperm to become embryos can truly be termed good quality.

Speaking of sperm, let's not forget about the other side of the equation! Even if you have an infinite number of quality eggs, it takes two to tango. The quality of the sperm can obviously have an impact on the future success of your eggs, too.

DOCTOR INSIGHT: "There is no good way to test whether the eggs that women have frozen are of good quality (have normal chromosomal makeup). The only way to know if the chromosomes are normal is to fertilize the egg with sperm, create an embryo and then biopsy the embryo and perform preimplantation genetic testing on the embryo. If the embryo has a normal number of chromosomes, then you know that the egg that it came from is also normal." - Dr. Diana Chavkin, HRC Fertility, Los Angeles

So, in short, it's currently impossible to know with any real certainty whether your eggs are good quality or not until you use them. Despite the unknowns, there are some indicators to help forecast the likelihood that one or more of your eggs will become healthy babies one day, metrics that you can use as a rule of thumb:

It depends on how old you are when you freeze your eggs, and how many eggs you freeze

There are other variables, too, such as your individual health and medical history, the practitioners' skills, the quality of the lab, and other lifestyle factors that positively or negatively affect the quality of the eggs retrieved.

The sooner you freeze, the higher the chance of a baby

Your response to ovarian stimulation medications could change from month-to-month, or with different treatment protocols, just as your own menstrual cycle can. As a result, the calculation is unique to each woman and impossible to accurately predict individually. However, as a rule of thumb, the quality and quantity of eggs you're likely to retrieve in your egg freezing cycle will decrease with each year older you become. In 2017, Harvard scientists created the world's first evidence-based model to help women and doctors gauge the likelihood of success by age, to assist in family-building planning. According to this model, assuming you have a normal ovarian reserve, one cycle of egg freezing at age 35 gives you an 80% likelihood of having a baby using those eggs, regardless of the age at which you use them, whereas if you freeze your eggs at age 40, you would need five cycles to have the same chance.[227] This is why doctors sometimes recommend multiple cycles of egg freezing to older women.

Note: You might be surprised to see that the number of mature eggs retrieved increases again in a woman's early 40s. Doctors report this can be the case with natural conception, too. Older mothers are more likely to ovulate more than one egg in a cycle and have twins, perhaps functioning as biology's "last hurrah." But despite this increase in eggs retrieved, the chances of them being good quality are low. This is why even if you retrieve two more eggs at age 41 than if you were 40, your chances of having a baby are still the same (25%).

Egg freezing prediction model, by age of freezing			
Age at freezing	Average number of mature eggs retrieved from one cycle	Percent chance of a live birth from one cycle	Number of cycles needed to have a ~75% chance of a live birth
≤35	14	80%	1
36	15	72%	1
37	12	56%	1
38	9	38%	2
39	9	33%	3
40	8	25%	4
41	10	25%	5
42	10	20%	5
≥43	7	10%	6

So, overall, the likelihood of your frozen eggs leading to a healthy baby in the future rests on both the quantity you freeze and the age at which you freeze them (which is indicative of the quality of the eggs.)

Although the unknowns and lack of certainty can feel frustrating, one way to think of it is to flip it on its head and focus on the certainties we *do* have: that each year older you get the likelihood of you conceiving a healthy child naturally *will* fall and if you do need IVF, the likelihood of you having a healthy baby using your younger frozen eggs would be greater than using your older fresh eggs.

The more eggs you freeze, the higher chance of a baby

The road from egg to baby is full of obstacles. Many things can prevent an egg from reaching the finish line, from the skill of the doctors managing the stimulation cycle, to the quality of the eggs retrieved, and even the laboratory environment. Basically, it's a numbers game. Here are just a few of the obstacles that your eggs must overcome (based on conservative estimates):

- **At freezing:** 15-20% of the eggs retrieved may not be mature enough to be frozen.[228]

- **At thawing:** 85-90% of eggs are likely to survive the egg freezing and thawing process.[229] However, according to Dr. Chavkin, if you freeze only good quality eggs then you'd have close to 100% thawing success but if you freeze immature and poor quality eggs then your chance of survival would be less.

- **At fertilization:** Not all of your previously frozen eggs will be successfully fertilized by sperm and effectively transformed into an embryo. According to doctors on our expert panel, the fertilization rate is between 70% to 80%, assuming that the sperm is of adequate quality.

- **At implantation:** Less than half of embryos resulting from your previously frozen eggs will successfully implant. This can range from 17-40% depending on the age you froze your eggs,[230] [231] [232] [233] which is roughly the same rate as fresh eggs of the same age.[234] Common health conditions such as endometriosis, obesity, and uterine fibroids can reduce the likelihood of implantation.[235] On the other hand, advancements in genetic testing, specifically preimplantation genetic screening (PGS), can increase implantation rates. That's because once all embryos are tested for quality, only the one(s) with the right number of chromosomes are implanted. This test does come at an additional cost ($3,000-$7,000) but could dramatically reduce the number of IVF cycles needed to achieve a successful pregnancy,[236] [237] especially if you were over 35 at the time of freezing. Not only that, but it can help reduce the devastating emotional impacts of failed implantation and miscarriage.

- **During pregnancy:** The miscarriage rate following assisted reproductive technology (ART) treatment is 15%, which is comparable to that following natural conception.[238]

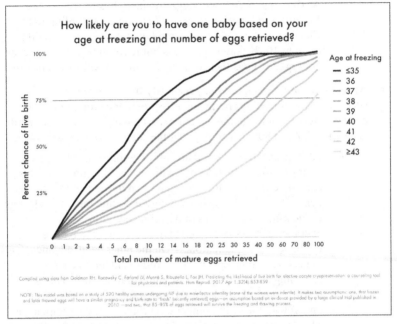

How likely are you to have one baby based on your age at freezing and number of eggs retrieved?

In other words, even a high-quality egg may not survive the journey to becoming a baby, which is why a higher number of frozen eggs increases your chances. Of course, good quality sperm is responsible for the other half of the pregnancy equation.

It depends on your "ovarian reserve"

There is not one universally agreed definition of this oft-cited phrase. But generally, ovarian reserve refers to our fertility potential based on the number and quality of eggs and our ovaries' capacity to respond to hormone signals from the brain to mature those eggs.[239] While every woman's ovarian reserve gradually decreases with age,[240] the rate at which it declines varies greatly from one of us to another, even if we're the same age from the start.[241] [242] The variance in the rate of ovarian reserve decline has been linked, in part, to how quickly the ovary itself is aging. For women with rapid rate of decline, this causes what is considered "early onset menopause," which has been linked to diabetes, cardiovascular diseases, neurological diseases, and even mortality.[243] [244] [245]

Having an idea what your ovarian reserve looks like can help you and your doctor predict how well your ovaries will respond to the hormones, and thus how many eggs you're likely to retrieve.[246] This is an important step in the process, as it will help you set your expectations.

Tests to determine the ovarian reserve have been somewhat of an evolving science and are still not 100% accurate. The most accurate predictor is still the most low-tech: your age.[247] However, reproductive authorities now agree that a blood test measuring anti-Mullerian hormone (AMH) levels in addition to your antral follicle counts (AFC) measured via pelvic ultrasound paints the most accurate picture of how you will respond to ovarian stimulation.[248] [249] AMH is a hormone produced by the cells that line follicles, so therefore the more follicles, the more AMH is produced. As such, doctors interpret higher AMH as reflecting higher ovarian reserve and greater fertility potential.

Blood tests that measure follicle stimulating hormone (FSH) as well as other ovarian substances like estradiol and inhibin B were once standard measures for ovarian reserve but are less commonly measured nowadays, because the results may fluctuate from month-to-month. They are not as reliable measures as AMH and AFC.[250] [251] [252] [253] [254] We'll discuss when and how to get these tests in Chapter 6, "Picking the Clinic."

DOCTOR INSIGHT: "To assess ovarian reserve or egg number doctors will definitely use age as a rough estimate to predict such a thing, but antral follicle count (AFC) and anti Mullerian hormone (AMH) are key. Both are often used together to predict ovarian reserve and fertility." - Dr. Diana Chavkin, HRC Fertility, Los Angeles

Still, there are no guarantees

Every healthcare provider should be upfront in telling you the facts and, if you feel like you're getting oversold and the facts are being glossed over, you don't have to go back. It's as simple as that. There are many wonderful and wise fertility doctors out there whom you can trust to give you the real facts, while also giving you options for your future, so don't settle for care from someone who isn't placing your best interests front and center. (More on how to pick a clinic later.)

Egg freezing gives you an extra chance of conceiving a biological child in the future, but we all need to keep our feet on the ground as there is actually no guarantee of being able to have a child from those frozen eggs in the future. It might not work. Natural conception should be the goal, with egg freezing representing a backup, not your life plan.

EXPERT INSIGHT: "With egg freezing, it is important to realize that we do not have the extensive outcomes data, (pregnancy rates most importantly) that we have generated with IVF over the past twenty years. We can make educated assumptions about the likelihood of success based on past cycles using cryopreserved eggs and embryos, but we will not have generated these numbers for quite a few years." - Dr. David Sable, Healthcare and Life Science Investor

Question 9: Does it matter how old I am when I go back to use my eggs?

There is no legal limit in the US

There is no legal age limit for having IVF in the US, nor is there a limit on the length of time that eggs can be stored. (Note that in some countries this is not the case - for instance, in the UK, there is currently an arbitrary storage limit of ten years, which campaigners are trying to have overturned.)

But there are some ethical limits to bear in mind

Some clinics limit the age at which a woman can undergo IVF with their own, fresh eggs because of the limited chance of success and, for much older women, the futility of it. There is also potentially some limit to how old you are when you can attempt pregnancy with your frozen eggs. The American Society for Reproductive Medicine (ASRM) believes that doctors should discourage women over 55 years old from having embryo transfers.[255] However, in practice, many fertility clinics have upper age limits (often around 45-50 years old) for embryo transfer. Some will go beyond this age, though.

There is no known biological limit

Doctors do not generally advocate attempting IVF (even with donor eggs from another woman, or using your own frozen eggs) beyond your late 40s, but as it currently stands, there is not enough definitive data to formulate a strict biological age limit that would prevent you from using your eggs in the future.

Theoretically, if you are healthy you could be any age when you use your eggs, because, if you recall, it's the age of the egg (fresh or frozen) that matters, not the age of the womb.[256] Despite this, there are medical implications for carrying a baby later in life, regardless of the age of the egg. Women pregnant at older ages are associated with higher rates of gestational diabetes, preeclampsia, cesarean delivery and premature babies with low birth weights. However, these risks vary widely, depending on the woman's health status, and increase with maternal age at delivery.[257][258] But, if you freeze your eggs at 35, whether you go back to use them at 38 or 43-years-old, your chances of conceiving would be just the same, notwithstanding general health concerns.[259]

There are reports of women conceiving using IVF and donor eggs well into their 50s, 60s and even at 70 in some countries, though it is rare.[260]

> **The world's oldest IVF mother**
> In 2019, a 78 year old woman in India delivered healthy twin girls who were conceived via IVF using donor eggs and her 74 year old husband's sperm. The couple reportedly married in 1962 and had been waiting 57 years to become parents. Previously, the oldest verified mother was a Spanish woman who gave birth to twins in 2006 age 66, then passed away age 69 after being diagnosed with cancer shortly after giving birth. She had IVF at a California clinic, having reportedly lied, telling them she was 55 years old.[261]

In addition, the amount of time your frozen eggs are stored does not affect the ability for them to be successfully thawed in the future, nor does it hinder the implantation rate or the pregnancy rate per warming cycle.[262] This should mean that storing your eggs for two years would merit the same results as storing them for 20 years.

There's not a great deal of research in this area, but a team of UK researchers looked at five years worth of data from London fertility clinics and found that, on average, women returned to use their frozen eggs at age 43.[263]

DOCTOR INSIGHT: "Many of my patients are unaware of the fact that even post-menopausal women can conceive with donor eggs or their previously frozen eggs." Dr. Carolyn Givens, Pacific Fertility Center, San Francisco

Question 10: Should I freeze eggs or embryos?

Embryo freezing is an established technique involving freezing your eggs once they have already been fertilized by sperm. This has some advantages and some drawbacks. If you are considering freezing embryos, there are some very important things to consider before doing so. The decision to freeze embryos comes with clinical, personal, and potentially legal ramifications that might be difficult to grapple with now but could save you a lot of trouble in the future.

In terms of the process, embryo freezing is exactly the same as egg freezing except that after your eggs are retrieved, they would be fertilized with sperm in a lab, which would hopefully continue to develop into embryos *before* they are frozen - essentially completing two-thirds of the process of a full IVF cycle. In an egg freezing cycle, you would only have completed the first third of the process, leaving fertilization until the time you want to use them.

Is the success rate better?

The biggest misconception about freezing embryos is the success rate. Because an embryo is more fully formed than an egg, it's considered less delicate. In the past, this equated to a higher likelihood that it would thaw correctly from its frozen state. However, with the development of the fast freezing technique called vitrification, thaw rates of eggs are almost exactly the same as embryos now - roughly 90% for eggs and 95% for embryos.

But, let's be clear, that doesn't mean your chances of achieving a successful live birth are five percent higher, it just means that embryos are a tiny bit more likely to make it to the next phase of the IVF process. And, the higher quality eggs that are frozen (i.e. if you freeze your eggs relatively young and maintain a healthy lifestyle), the more likely those thaw rates could be just as good, if not higher than that of embryos. What all that being said, if you are freezing eggs later in life and you have a known "sperm source" (that's not a great term, is it? But it's the politically correct way of saying person or donor with whom you definitely want to make babies in the future!), then even this small bit of an advantage might make sense to you. This is something to discuss with your doctor. Whichever option you choose, prepare for the fact that only a percentage of your eggs will actually produce embryos, and even those might not implant successfully.

DOCTOR PERSPECTIVE: "I always review the tradeoffs of freezing eggs versus embryos. In general, I counsel women that freezing eggs provides her with more flexibility and the outcomes are similar to freezing embryos."
- Dr. Meera Shah, Nova IVF, Mountain View

DOCTOR PERSPECTIVE: "When considering freezing eggs vs. freezing embryos, the choice comes down to your risk tolerance, relationship status, and desire for optionality in the future. By freezing embryos, you are committing to a single sperm source – your eggs can never be 'unfertilized' so you lose all flexibility. What you gain however, is an increase in efficiency of the entire process. Freezing and subsequently thawing eggs typically results in a 10-20% attrition in the number of viable eggs. By eliminating this stage of the IVF process, you will have a greater number of eggs to fertilize and a higher probability of success. Embryos also have the benefit of knowing how many of your eggs developed well. Thus you have more certainty on the outcome, good or bad." – Dr. Peter Klatsky, Spring Fertility, San Francisco

What are the benefits of freezing embryos?

Arguably the biggest benefit of freezing embryos is simply having more data to work with. With egg freezing, you want to get as many eggs as possible in the *hopes* that at least one of them will become a healthy baby. In the case of freezing embryos, you'll be able to get a much better idea how many of those eggs are actually good quality. If it's not a satisfactory number, you could then plan accordingly - let's say move forward your plans for trying naturally or do another cycle of ovarian stimulation right away.

Keep in mind that not all of your eggs will become embryos. And from there, you can choose to test your remaining embryos for chromosomal abnormalities. So, by the time all that is said and done, you'll have a pretty good idea what your chances of success will be in the future. Didn't get the number of embryos you wanted? Now you can make a more informed decision as to whether or not to do another cycle, especially in your more fertile years.

DOCTOR PERSPECTIVE: "Whenever I speak with a patient that is married or in a seriously committed relationship, but they are just not ready to start a family, I always recommend consideration of banking fertilized eggs – embryo banking. They survive thawing at a slightly higher rate and can be tested for their chromosomes at the time of freezing so they are so much closer to being a baby." -Dr. Carolyn Givens, Pacific Fertility Center, San Francisco

DOCTOR PERSPECTIVE: "Freezing eggs definitely gives you reproductive autonomy over freezing embryos. However, if you definitely know you are going to have children with a particular partner but are not ready now then freezing embryos may give you a bit more reassurance. Meaning you have a better idea of what you have in the bank. If you freeze 10 eggs you don't really know how many of them will turn into embryos. But if you have 10 frozen, you are a lot further down the path toward pregnancy and so your safety net is a bit stronger. It also lets you know earlier and at a younger age if you should do more cycles. Meaning if you got 10 eggs you may feel great about that. But what if those 10 eggs were only destined to become 1 embryo? Well then if you got to that embryo stage, you likely would consider another cycle before you let another five years go by. But if those 10 eggs resulted in 10 embryos then you'd feel more comfortable stopping there. With frozen eggs there is just more unknown when compared to frozen embryos." - Dr. Diana Chavkin, HRC Fertility, Los Angeles

What are the potential drawbacks?

There is far more potential for ethical dilemmas around their storage and fate (some people and countries have religious or moral objections or laws) and issues surrounding "ownership." Decisions over the fate of stored embryos can also lead to major disagreements or legal disputes, particularly in the case of divorce or separation.[264]

Ultimately, once your egg is fertilized by sperm, it will always carry those genetics - there's no going back. So, your relationship with the owner of that sperm (and potential co-owner of the embryo) needs to be really clear.

Let's take a few examples. Perhaps you're in a new but promising relationship, or a steady long-term relationship, perhaps you're even married, freezing embryos can seem like an exciting way to solidify your future family goals together. But what if something happens to either one of you or your relationship before you'd want to use them? And what if those embryos turned out to be your only chance of having your own biological child? This is very important to consider in case of a breakup, divorce or even the untimely death of your partner. It's safe to assume that you don't go into a relationship thinking any of these awful things will happen but it's good to be realistic about any eventualities, as uncomfortable as they may be. In one cautionary tale, a couple from Arizona chose to freeze embryos before one of them, Ruby, underwent chemotherapy and radiation treatment for breast cancer. Years later, at age 37, Ruby's marriage fell apart. During the divorce proceedings, she requested to use her embryos because it was probably her only chance at having her own biological children; however, her soon-to-be-ex-husband rejected the request, as he no longer wishes to have children with her.[265]

In another high profile case, Modern Family actress Sofia Vergara has been entrenched in a long legal battle over the rights to her frozen embryos. In this case, her ex-husband wants to use them with the help of a surrogate. There are undeniable political components underlying this legal debate, which are rooted in the battle over reproductive freedoms. Vergara's former husband expressed his opinion in a New York Times op-ed piece: "Shouldn't a man who is willing to take on all parental responsibilities be similarly entitled to bring his embryos to term even if the woman objects? These are issues that, unlike abortion, have nothing to do with the rights over one's own body, and everything to do with a parent's right to protect the life of his or her unborn child."[266]

Each US state approaches their handling of these cases differently. Most often, courts weigh in support of the person that does not want the embryos used; however, at least in Arizona, courts are leaning towards the person that intends to "help the embryos develop to birth."[267] There's no really clear legal structure, though contracting carefully in advance with the help of a lawyer might be helpful. The point is that, when you look at these cases, it makes you realize you have to be *really* sure that linking that particular sperm to your eggs (which could one day represent your only shot at becoming a Mom) is the right idea, especially if you wait to use them past your most fertile years. And, if anything were to happen to your partner, it's worth asking yourself if you'd still want to use those embryos, particularly if you had a new partner on the scene.

It's a really complex thing, because you're dealing with a big blank where the future sits, and none of us really know what curveballs lie ahead however happy we might feel now. Because of the legal and emotional risks as well as the limitations placed on your reproductive autonomy, many doctors recommend seeing a couples counselor before following through with your decision.

"Before my second round of egg freezing, my partner and I talked about whether to freeze eggs or embryos. He was open to embryo freezing, but I decided to freeze eggs for a few different reasons. The first was as it felt like the decision that protected my independence and empowered me as a women the most in the long run. Despite the fact that I'm in a committed, loving relationship with a person that I hope to grow old with, the reality is that relationships end, people get divorced and people die. Second, although as a couple we are ready to commit to each other, we're not necessarily ready to commit to having a child together and we were suddenly confronted with all kinds of ethical questions that we were not ready to answer. For example, if we decide to go our separate ways or one of us dies, who gets to decide what happens with the embryo given that both sets of our DNA are at play here? How do we feel about donating the embryos or discarding them? We decided that as soon as we were ready to commit to having children together we would freeze an embryo(s) then, taking further proactive steps towards family planning." - Erika, 37

EXPERT PERSPECTIVE: "I recently met with a couple that had been together for a long time. She was ready to get married and have babies, but he wasn't. She was 39, so it made sense for her to freeze her eggs in the meantime, but when she brought up freezing embryos, he didn't want to commit. I referred them to a couples' counselor, which I think has been really helpful for them. Because of her age, she decided to freeze her eggs now and then do an embryo freezing cycle later if the counseling goes well." - Peggy Orlin, Marriage and Family Therapist Specializing in Infertility, Pacific Fertility Center, San Francisco

Is there a cost difference?

An important thing to factor into this is the relative cost of both options, too. If you choose to freeze embryos, you'll pay more up front to have your eggs fertilized and genetically tested, a cost that you will bear whether you use them or not. On the other hand, if you are able to get all the embryo testing done up front and discover that you have to do another cycle, this could save you from doing multiple rounds of IVF using your older, fresh eggs down the line, if you do need to use them. Many of these considerations will be more or less pertinent depending on the age you are now, when you would want to use them and how confident you are that you'll use them in the future.

Question 11: Are there any special considerations I should factor in?

How is my general health?

Some medical conditions - past or current - could put your fertility at risk or mean you have more difficulty conceiving than most women your age. For example, chlamydia is the most common cause of infertility in women, as the infection carries with it considerable risk of spreading to fallopian tubes.[268] For some women with these types of reproductive issues, egg freezing could represent a better chance of conception down the line since you may need IVF anyway. In essence, you may want to get the "first step" of IVF (ovarian stimulation) out of the way early and freeze your eggs while they are as young as possible. If you are affected by a reproductive health condition, this is something to discuss with your doctor.

One potentially limiting factor in determining whether or not a clinic might deem you a "candidate" for egg freezing is you are severely overweight. Most clinics have a BMI cut-off for egg freezing because of the increased health risks for overweight women going under anesthesia.

DOCTOR INSIGHT: "Our clinic's BMI cut-off is 40+ but other clinics' are usually slightly higher. The main problem is that obese women can present health problems and, as they have a greater tendency to sleep apnea, if they have a respiratory arrest, it may be very difficult to intubate them. I have never had this happen with an egg freezing or IVF patient but I have seen it at a C-section. Very scary." - Dr. Carolyn Givens, Pacific Fertility Center, San Francisco

Did my mom go through early menopause?

This might seem like a weird question, but this can provide a prediction of when you're likely to go through it yourself, as there seems to be some genetic link. Menopause is effectively the culmination of the continuous process of ovarian aging,[269] so, if your mother's ovaries aged faster than average that could be important information to pass to your fertility doctor. So, what's normal? The wider range for menopause is anything from 40-60 years old,[270] [271] but the average age for a woman to get her last period is 51 years old. That doesn't necessarily mean she can conceive up to that point - ovulation is likely to be very irregular for some years before this. If your mother experienced menopause a lot earlier than around 50 years old, especially under 40, that's worth flagging up to your specialist during your medical consultation. Interestingly, there's a theory that it takes 6 years from the first sign of menstrual cycle irregularities (for instance, shortening by a few days[272]) to reach menopause - something to note for when we all eventually reach that stage.[273] [274]

What if I've been diagnosed with a "low" or "diminished" ovarian reserve?

If you're over the age of 37, your blood test indicated lower levels of AMH and your AFC scan showed fewer follicles, your doctor might have talked to you about being a "poor responder" to the ovarian stimulation hormones that is typical of women with a diminished ovarian reserve. Before you freak out, rest assured that many women with low follicle counts can still successfully conceive, as long as their eggs are of high enough quality. A study measured the ovarian reserves (i.e. the number of follicles remaining in the ovaries) of 750 women from ages 30 to 44 who had no history of infertility and found that women with a lower egg count were just as likely to get pregnant as those with a high egg count. Without any correlation between ovarian reserve and fertility, this leaves egg quality as the primary determinant of a whether those pregnancies resulted in live births or miscarriage.

So, how might this news shape your decision on whether or not to freeze your eggs? In our opinion, it's a bit of a catch-22. Your doctor might advise you not to freeze because you won't retrieve many eggs, and even risk having the cycle cancelled altogether because the ovaries respond so poorly. On the other hand, your ovarian reserve will continue to decline so even freezing a few of your younger (and likely higher quality) eggs is better than nothing, if you can afford to, of course. One thing to note is that you may still be pretty fertile, you might just need to be open to doing more cycles.

What if I've missed periods, or they are very light?

Light or irregular periods should not be an indicator in and of itself that you won't respond well to ovarian stimulation medications. Going on or off birth control, or switching methods, can cause changes in your flow or the length of your period. Sometimes women even miss a period during stressful times, like grief or a major deadline. Missed or light periods could also be caused by over exercising or not eating enough rather than being a direct indication of your fertility arc. It's best to mention any missed or lighter/heavier than usual periods to your doctor - your consultation is a great time to do that. Some women approaching their late 30s do have less regular periods, as fertility starts to reduce. This could be the start of your body's slow transition to perimenopause, which is normal and natural.

While your regularity and lightness of your period are data inputs, the length of your menstrual cycle might actually be a more important metric when it comes to fertility. A study found women under 30 who were diagnosed with premature ovarian insufficiency (a condition when a woman's ovaries stop working normally before she is 40) actually continued to have their periods regularly and as normal without change *except* for their cycle length shortening.

Tracking your menstrual cycle can also help you get a good handle on what baseline "normal" is for you and if that starts to change - there are many tools, digital or otherwise, that can help you with this. Check out the resources and reviews on our website for more guidance on what options are available.

Doctors can only really diagnose whether any menstrual cycle changes might have implications for your egg freezing cycle or for your wider fertility by analyzing test results, such as the test for AMH levels. So, even if you monitor your period and notice changes, it's important not to jump to any conclusions about your fertility on your own.

Do I have to take birth control pills before treatment?

The main benefit to taking birth control pills prior your egg freezing cycle is that it allows for better scheduling. Basically, patients and doctors are both better able to plan when it's going to happen. This is especially useful if you are traveling for treatment or if you have PCOS - it's harder for doctors to plan and manage the stimulation cycles of women with PCOS without putting them on the pill, as they often have irregular cycles. There are some studies that flag concerns in using birth control for potentially low responders, or older women, so doctors may avoid pre-treatment in these cases. Ask your doctor about the risks and reasoning if she or he has suggested using birth control pills as part of your treatment plan, or if you are already on hormonal contraceptives and have questions about how that fits in with the cycle.

DOCTOR PERSPECTIVE: "Birth control pills may be used as an adjunct to prepare the ovaries for many patients, depending on the protocol their physicians recommend. This is a common preparation treatment particularly for women with PCOS or good ovarian reserve. In these cases, birth control pills will 'prime' the ovaries and synchronize the egg follicles to more closely regulate their growth. As a general rule some providers, including myself, will tend away from birth control pills if a patient has a low to moderate ovarian reserve." – Dr. Peter Klatsky, Spring Fertility, San Francisco

What if I have an IUD?

Having an intrauterine device (IUD) does not appear to impact the results of an egg freezing cycle.[275] Even if you don't have period because of the IUD, doctors can often start your stimulation at any point (doctors often refer to this as a "random start,") which still yields the same results overall as traditional approach. And you don't even need to take it out!

What if I've been diagnosed with endometriosis?

Endometriosis, a painful condition in which womb tissue grows outside the womb, can cause infertility. For reasons that doctors don't understand very well, the endometrium (womb lining cells) accumulate inside the pelvis where they can cause scarring on the ovaries, fallopian tubes, bladder bowel and rectum, damaging them. Although endometriosis can be removed during surgery to help improve fertility, this cannot always be done completely.

Research indicates that 30% to 50% of women diagnosed with endometriosis struggle with infertility.[276] But this reproductive issue is challenging to identify in the first place, taking an average of four years before a woman receives the correct diagnosis.[277] The chronic, non-infectious inflammation can increase a woman's potential for diminished ovarian reserve and decrease egg quality and egg quantity,[278] which is why egg freezing presents as an option before the condition gets worse.

DOCTOR INSIGHT: "*We don't advise women with endometriosis early enough to freeze their eggs. When a woman is given this diagnosis, she should be immediately counseled as to preserving fertility. If there is a family history of endometriosis, she is more likely to have that diagnosis as well.*" *- Dr. Aimee Eyvazzadeh, Private Practice Physician, San Ramon*

DOCTOR INSIGHT: "*Endometriosis can decrease egg quality. Surgery to remove endometriosis on the ovary can often compromise egg supply. Some studies suggest that nearly half of all infertile couples have endometriosis, therefore it is a high risk factor for infertility.*" *- Dr. Meera Shah, Nova IVF, Mountain View*

DOCTOR INSIGHT: "*Some women may want to freeze eggs before having surgery, especially if they are at risk of having one or both ovaries removed.*" *- Dr. Lynn Westphal, Kindbody and Stanford University School of Medicine*

DOCTOR INSIGHT: "*Because endometriosis is a progressive disease, the younger a woman with endometriosis is, the less endometriosis she will have compared to later in life - and less endo means a better egg number and quality. So, to save some of her eggs from the influence of the endo it would be a good idea for someone with severe and worsening endo to think about freezing eggs perhaps at an earlier age than someone without endo.*" *- Dr. Diana Chavkin, HRC Fertility, Los Angeles*

DOCTOR INSIGHT: "*For some women with endometriosis and chronic pelvic pain, the best treatment option for pain (after medications fail) is surgery to remove endometriosis from the pelvis. When this includes removing endometriosis cysts from the ovaries, there is a known risk of reducing ovarian reserve (number of follicles i.e. eggs) – which can impact future fertility or even reduce time to menopause slightly in some cases. Egg freezing prior to surgery on the ovaries may be one way to prevent associated potential decline in fertility. (the same is true for an assortment of ovarian surgeries for other cysts like dermoids).*" *- Dr. Eleni Greenwood Jaswa, University of California, San Francisco*

DOCTOR INSIGHT: "I would say that if a woman has endometriosis, she has probably had that diagnosis made because of her symptoms of pain. Although it is less commonly done in recent times, if the pain is very severe, at some point she may have to opt to have definitive surgery, i.e. hysterectomy or oophorectomy. Also, even if pain is not an issue, because endometriosis is commonly associated with infertility, and it has been shown that IVF is the best treatment for endometriosis-related infertility, that woman may end up needing to do IVF anyway in the future in order to conceive. So doing egg freezing sooner than later would make the success of eventual IVF better because of having younger eggs to work with. So, if anything, a woman with endometriosis has more reasons to consider egg freezing." - Dr. Carolyn Givens, Pacific Fertility Center, San Francisco

Overall, most doctors counsel that in cases of severe endometriosis (where the physical remaining tissue of the ovaries is greatly reduced, with severe reduction of the function of the ovaries), egg freezing is a suitable solution. An AMH test can be used to determine the ovarian function and if the function is severely reduced, then egg freezing might be advised. However, with mild endometriosis it would usually be advised there is no need for egg freezing for that reason.

What if I've been diagnosed with polycystic ovary syndrome (PCOS)?

If you've been diagnosed with PCOS, you should be aware of a few things regarding egg freezing. First, the good news: you might retrieve more eggs and you might pay less for medication! That's because ovaries are likely, on average, to be more sensitive to the hormones than women without PCOS, so your dosing might be lower or your stimulation cycle shorter. The less good news is: because of the way your ovaries respond to the hormones, you might be at more risk than other women of your ovaries getting over stimulated and developing a (thankfully rare) condition called ovarian hyperstimulation syndrome (OHSS).[279] It might also be the case that fewer of the eggs you have retrieved are considered good quality/mature enough to freeze, but given you're likely to get more, on a percentage basis, the net result is thought to be similar to a woman without PCOS.[280] So this is unlikely to be a concern unless you are very overweight as well as having PCOS - there's some research that suggests in that case you may risk poorer egg and embryo quality than women with PCOS who are not overweight.[281] [282] (A great reason to stick to the healthy diet principles in Part Two, if you think you need some motivation in that area.)

PCOS is considered the most common reproductive disorder for women under 50, affecting an estimated 5–15% of women worldwide.[283] Symptoms - caused by hormone imbalances - include irregular or no periods, excessive hair growth on the face, chest, back or butt, weight struggles, thinning hair and hair loss from the head, oily skin or acne, sleep problems and fatigue.

PCOS falls into the category of "ovulatory disorder" because the hormonal imbalances can lead to your eggs not developing properly, which can make it harder to get pregnant. Instead of a mature egg being released in ovulation, your eggs may be arrested at a small, immature stage, leading to many of them remaining in your follicles and resembling little cysts on your ovaries - this is what the "polycystic" bit of the name refers to.

Luckily, the power of modern medicine can kick in! In an egg freezing cycle, the fertility medications will stimulate your ovaries to keep pushing your eggs through the various stages of maturity, when they might have otherwise stopped naturally. The takeaway is that having PCOS isn't a deal breaker or maker in your egg freezing decision, but you should be aware that the process and the outcome might be a little different from other women.

Question 12: What has led me to explore egg freezing?

There's an obvious answer: wanting to preserve your fertility. But looking more deeply, this can be a difficult question for women to answer, as it involves unpacking a number of different inputs, not all of them personal and not all of them immediately clear. According to some less tolerant media outlets, the stereotypical "egg freezing woman" is a career-hungry, glass-ceiling smasher, liable to hiss if she encounters a baby en route from the boardroom to the wine bar.[284] We don't know about you, but that really doesn't capture a full or accurate picture of our lives (except for maybe the wine bar). Deciding to freeze your eggs is a personal decision, but it's also one that's inextricable linked to the wider social context. Understanding why other women decided to do it can give you insights that can help you make sense of the decision in front of you, as well as clarity on the bigger picture. Each woman's individual reasons for egg freezing are nuanced and informed by a mixed bag of personal, societal, and structural circumstances that aren't easy to generalize.

It's not the "right time" to start a family

Contrary to how it can feel when you're single and *could not be more ready* to mingle, the "right time" is not all about finding the right partner, for both men and women.[285] Research shows that even women in relationships choose to freeze their eggs because they are "just not ready for kids yet."[286] For many women, both in relationships or not, being "ready" for kids means that certain (self-defined) life conditions need to be in place before they would choose parenthood. Some of these conditions were found to include things like having a stable job, sound finances and/or having a home in a child-friendly area.[287] For many women and men, these life conditions aren't merely preferences, but prerequisites.

"My boyfriend and I are pretty sure we want to have kids together someday, but we are SO not in a place in our lives financially where we would even consider it. I know that egg freezing is expensive, but the cost of having a child is exponentially higher. I want to be a good parent and for me that can only happen once I have time and financial stability." - Jennie, 35

My partner isn't ready for parenthood

For many women, having a partner to co-parent with is an important consideration when choosing whether or not to have a child, albeit not a necessity (the number of women who are single mothers by choice (or "SMC") is growing.)[288] Even for those in relationships, co-parenting is not automatically on the cards. Women get a lot of bashing, but one study found that many women in relationships who froze their eggs did so because their partner would not commit to fatherhood.[289] This is perhaps in part due to men being even less informed about the impact of age on fertility than women are.

"I've been with my boyfriend for years now and he's made it clear that he does want to start a family with me someday, but that seems to be on his own time, not mine. It's not like I'm going to be able to have kids forever! He hasn't even proposed and it's not something I feel like I can bring up yet again...egg freezing seems like the only option." – Hilary, 36

I haven't found the right partner

Despite the rise in "SMCs," the majority preference of women is still to raise a child with a life partner. That could be for many different reasons, not the least of which is economics – many women we spoke to said that they felt raising a child in their city was something you could only do with two salaries. 85% of the women from a Yale University study on egg freezing were single and many of these women said they froze their eggs because they didn't have a suitable partner with whom to raise a child.

What's most interesting from the Yale research is that, in contrast to the old stereotype, only 1.5% of the women said they froze their eggs for directly career-related purposes.[290] [291]

It's not as if the single women in this study had no interest in relationships when they were younger - the majority of them said that throughout their college and career-building years they had been looking for the right person they could one day start a family with, but it just hadn't happened.

"It's not like I haven't been trying to find a decent guy to date. I'm just not willing to settle. For me, having kids is more about starting a family with the right person. I'd rather do it right the first time rather than end up divorced with kids like my parents did." - Bonnie, 38

DOCTOR INSIGHT: "Most women I see for a consultation for egg freezing are considering it because they are currently not in a relationship and have a strong desire to have children in the future. I also see many women who are in serious relationships but want to delay childbearing to pursue higher education, career aspirations, or have experienced a recent personal hardship." - Dr. Meera Shah, Nova IVF, Mountain View

Single women in another study also said they froze their eggs because they knew they were running out of time to become mothers, but wanted to avoid so called "panic partnering:" a frantic decision to settle down (emphasis on the "settle") in an unsuitable relationship in order to have a biological child before the biological clock stops ticking.[292] The women from this study said that egg freezing gave them more time to find the right partner and avoid later regrets that they had settled down with the wrong guy. The life phase of "waiting for the right partner" is now so widespread it's become a new life stage for some women in their thirties and forties; there's even a term for it: "otherhood."[293]

That said, there are many routes to "otherhood." Some of the single women who froze eggs had previously *thought* they had found a life partner, but found themselves in unforeseen relationship issues, divorce (17%) or breakups (12%). Unsurprisingly, the women described these breakups as "traumatic," partly because they had spent most of their fertile years in that relationship, only to part ways with the men with whom they had previously planned to start a family. Amazingly, several of the women included the cost of egg freezing in their divorce settlements! [294]

DOCTOR INSIGHT: "A large proportion of my patients come to see me for egg freezing after a breakup or divorce." - Dr. Diana Chavkin, HRC Fertility, Los Angeles

So why are women in their fertile years seemingly finding it harder to find an acceptable partner who is willing to start a family? One theory is that many women have expectations about their partner's education and income that limit the pool of prospective partners.

In the US, college-educated women now significantly outnumber college-educated men: there are currently three million fewer of those men than women in their prime reproductive years, aged 22 to 39.[295] This means that college-educated women increasingly face a smaller pool of equally educated men with whom to start a family.

In one study, some women who froze their eggs said not being able to find a guy with their own level of education and earning power meant they had to "settle." For them, finding a partner with a similar background - namely, college-educated, or professional, often with advanced degrees or high earnings - were just really hard to find.[296] What they are describing is essentially a kind of dating glass ceiling for men. Their preferences run contrary to demographic shifts in the US - and the mismatch has obvious consequences.

In addition, men are also waiting longer to start families. Studies suggest the vast majority of men want and expect to become fathers. They aspire to have at least two children and are just as concerned as women about the timing and planning of them.[297] [298] Whether it's finishing college, establishing a career or finding "the one," both men and women say that it just has to be at the right time in life.[299] [300] [301] [302] [303]

The biggest discrepancy between men and women seems to be that the "right time" to have kids comes later for men than it does for women. For women, the "right time" is heavily regulated by the biological clock. While this runs in the background as a consistent reminder of the reproductive expiration date, the motivation to have kids really kicks in once certain life goals and milestones have been reached – things like financial stability or finding the right partner.[304]

While men also say they want to push back parenthood in order to achieve certain life goals, they differ from women in that they find it more important to have a few years of freedom before facing the sacrifices in time, flexibility, freedom, and career opportunities that fatherhood entails.[305] And perhaps the biggest difference is that men don't feel as constrained by their biological clock, which is why they don't often see their age as a limitation when it comes to fatherhood.[306] [307] Research indicates that the age-related constraints men do feel are informed by the desire to be an active father and to have their kids grow up in time for them to enjoy early retirement or so-called "second youth."[308]

"Of course I want to be a dad! Having a family has always been really important to me. I'm enjoying my life right now, dating and working hard. I just don't see the need to rush into anything." - Joe, 36

"My dad was the coach of my little league team and was always really involved in whatever sport I was playing. That's something I want to do for my kids one day." - Jeff, 32

Men's concept of the "right time" does not take into account their own biological clock: what many men don't realize is that sperm quality and quantity are thought to deteriorate around age 40.[309] [310] But, according to one of our Expert Panelists, Dr. Paul Turek, a noted male fertility specialist, the timeline of reduced male fertility potential "is more of an hourglass than a clock." In other words, fertility in men decreases much more gradually and less dramatically than in women. The most pronounced change in semen quality with advancing paternal age is lower sperm motility. Fewer sperm can mean a longer time to pregnancy.[311]

And older men are more likely to have miscarriages or babies with neurological diseases like schizophrenia.[312] [313] In fact, studies have shown that babies fathered by men over 55 years old have over four times the relative risk of having autism compared to fathers younger than 30. Scientists believe this stems from the fact that aging sperm is more likely to develop mutations.[314] In Dr. Turek's view, "the quality control machinery is getting older and wears down." Still, the changes in terms of infertility are still smaller than those in women.

It's not only an individual man's biological clock that we should start talking about: some scientists have also found evidence that suggests sperm counts have noticeably declined worldwide in the last century. One Danish study claims that the average sperm count has declined by more than 50% since 1973 and shows no sign of leveling off.[315] Despite the headlines splashed around on this topic, it's worth noting that the evidence is not conclusive and more research is needed.

If you have a partner and you're discussing when the "right time" might be, bear in mind that not only are men generally unaware of their own reproductive limitations, but they also overestimate a woman's fertility in her thirties.[316 317 318 319 320] Studies show that men also tend to overestimate the likelihood that assisted reproduction technologies like IVF would work and give them a child.[321 322 323 324 325 326 327] This is all a long way of saying that conflicting timelines can lead to feelings of deep frustration between partners,[328] so talking openly with your partner (or future partner) is important, using the actual facts and recognizing both of your emotional and personal preferences.

To gain a feeling of fertility freedom

For some women, egg freezing can be a decisive, empowering step that offers some security and insurance for the future and the *feeling* of taking the reins in their own lives.

"After I froze my eggs, I felt like a massive weight had been lifted off my shoulders. I know it's not guaranteed to work but knowing I've done everything I can has been a huge relief." - Gwen, 35

"I felt like a failure. Like I failed at my relationship, at being desirable as "mother material," like I failed at giving my parents a grandchild and failed to keep up with my friends. When I started looking into egg freezing, it felt like a way of getting back a bit of control, of making decisions about my own future and of realizing the reason I even can do this is because I am independent and successful." - Celia, 37

Because it's hard to combine parenthood and building a career

Women are accepted in the workplace, and we're finally moving our way up on the equality totem pole. But doesn't it seem like just when you get to the point in your career where you can finally be cleared of your school debt, the alarm bells start ringing from your biological clock? This is just one of many personal and systemic issues that pose conflict between parenthood and a career. When you look at the facts, "having it all" seems like nothing short of a pipe dream.

First, a career provides the obvious benefit of making money. For women, the financial opportunity grows with every year without children. In fact, studies show that delaying motherhood leads to a substantial increase in earnings of nine percent per year of delay.[329]

And even if or when you decide to have kids, the workplace is simply not outfitted for the demands of motherhood. As of 2018, the US is one of only three countries around the world without a national policy guaranteeing paid maternity leave. The benefits of paid maternity leave are far from trivial: a study found that the infants of women who did not receive it experienced almost double the odds of being re-hospitalized and double the chance of being re-hospitalized themselves within a year or two postpartum.[330]

And even after a child gets to the age when a woman no longer needs to provide basic care for an infant, such as breastfeeding, the conflict between career and motherhood doesn't seem to get much better. According to a Pew research study, 39% of women say that they have had to take "a significant amount of time off work" in order to take care of their children, versus only 24% of working fathers. As such, 42% of women said they've had to reduce their work hours to take care of the kids compared to only 28% of fathers.[331]

I'm unsure if I ever want kids

For women, single or in a relationship, who just aren't sure if they want kids, egg freezing can mean less worry that they might change their minds or regret the decision in the future when it might be too late.

"I always thought I'd have kids, but when I saw my friends with theirs, it made me really quickly realize that's just not the path for me. My husband, career, hobbies and dog are the perfect balance in my life. But I want to make sure I don't have any regrets when I'm in my forties." - Karen, 25

"It's been three years since I got divorced and I have a five year old son. I don't know if it's realistic to have more kids. I haven't dated at all and I would be really worried about rocking the boat for my son. But my company pays for egg freezing, so I'm going to do it just in case I meet someone great in the future and he wants a family of his own. I know I'm really lucky to have the option." - Berenice, 35

I want to prevent regret of <u>not</u> freezing

If it turns out that a woman needs her eggs and she didn't freeze them when she had the chance, she may blame herself. For some women it's less a case of believing egg freezing to be an insurance policy in and of itself, and more the case of insuring against her own potential future regret.[332]

I want to preserve my fertility before cancer treatment or radiation therapy

Anywhere from 20-70% of people who undergo cancer treatment will be left infertile by chemotherapy or radiation treatment.[333] Such treatments are known as "gonadotoxic" treatments because of the damage they can cause to the immature and growing follicles within the ovaries. If you are facing this kind of treatment, egg freezing might be a possibility and an opportunity to preserve your eggs. If having babies feels like the furthest thing from your mind, given everything on your plate, it's worth noting that for many women the desire to have children actually increased after surviving a cancer diagnosis.[334]

As you weigh your options, it's important to note that in the case of radiation therapy, the negative impact on your fertility is influenced by a few factors. First, where you receive the treatment on your body - radiation near the pelvic region seems to be the most damaging for fertility. Second, the cumulative dosage of the treatment. And lastly, your age at the time of treatment. Because, as we've discussed, the older you are, the fewer follicles you have to begin with. While there is still a chance you'll be able to conceive after radiation therapy, these factors could potentially place you in a pre-menopausal state.[335] In the case of chemotherapy, a similar outcome can occur in which your resting follicles are permanently damaged.[336] The most destructive chemotherapies include alkylating chemotherapies, such as cyclophosphamide, busulfan, melphalan procarbazine, and chemotherapeutic combinations that include alkylating chemotherapies.[337]

It should come as no surprise that having to grapple with a cancer diagnosis is already upsetting, which can only be made worse by the potential of future infertility, and having to decide whether or not to proceed with egg freezing. One bit of good news is that taking the time to freeze your eggs prior to chemotherapy will not delay the start of treatment.[338] This is thanks to a technique known as "random-start" ovarian stimulation, which means you won't need to wait for your next period. What you probably won't have time for is emotional recovery in between. For this reason, among others, you could be more at risk of experiencing depression and anxiety.[339] So, in anticipation of this challenging journey, it is recommended that you get a referral to a counselor, whether or not you decide to freeze your eggs.[340][341]

Despite a recent push for insurance companies to cover egg freezing for cancer patients, the current reality is that most of them do not.[342] This is no different to many healthy women considering egg freezing, except there are additional financial curveballs to anticipate: let's say further cancer treatment requires a hysterectomy and you cannot carry your frozen eggs or embryos yourself. Can you also afford the cost of a surrogate? Another unfortunate truth is that egg freezing won't be able to reverse all the potential damage caused to your reproductive system including the reproductive organs necessary for you to carry a pregnancy to term and the disruption of key reproductive hormones.[343]

Although egg freezing will not be the right path for all cancer patients, if you are of reproductive age and your future fertility could be compromised by medical treatment, make sure to have a discussion with your oncologist (or seek a referral to a fertility doctor) about your future fertility options.

DOCTOR INSIGHT: "Many cancers, most notably breast cancer, affect reproductive age women. With an expedited referral to a fertility specialist, a woman can undergo an egg freezing cycle in two weeks, without impacting her cancer treatment. As cancer treatments advance, more women are surviving their disease and living longer. Freezing eggs gives these women hope and a will to fight their cancer. This has been one of the most rewarding aspects of my job." - Dr. Meera Shah, Nova IVF, Mountain View

I'm gay, bi or in a same sex partnership

About five percent of American women consider themselves LGBT and the figure is even higher for women under age 40.[344] If that includes you and you know you one day want to have a genetic child, there are options such as at-home artificial insemination with a disposable syringe (i.e. the "turkey baster" method) or having sex with a guy (which may not sound like a super appealing option.) At-home artificial insemination has around the same success rate as intercourse. But, if it's not the right time yet, or, if you want to have a baby with a partner and think you'd like one of you to provide the eggs and the other to carry the baby in the future, egg freezing can help you to preserve your fertility potential until the time is right.

If you choose to use your eggs in the future, donor sperm would be used to fertilize the egg (in a petri dish) and the embryo would be implanted inside you or your chosen gestational mother in the hope of pregnancy.

The benefit is the same as it is for straight women: rather than going through an ovarian stimulation cycle at the point at which you are ready for a child (and retrieving older eggs), you could use your younger, better quality frozen eggs and skip straight to the embryo transfer stage.

The main disadvantage in freezing early rather than doing "fresh" IVF is that there will be additional storage costs involved. On the other hand, you might need fewer cycles of IVF because younger eggs have a higher chance of success.

"I've spent the last couple of years figuring out my sexuality and coming out to my friends and family. I've always wanted a big family and I know I want biological kids. It makes sense to me to freeze my eggs now if I will end up going through this in the future when I'm older anyway. I sold my car, took on some extra work and I'm using a payment plan to cover the rest." - Lex, 28

Because I'm undergoing gender reassignment

People preparing for transition may sometimes want to take steps to preserve their fertility before beginning hormone replacement therapy. Egg freezing can be a particularly strange and difficult thing for a person assigned female at birth, but transitioning, to go through: before taking testosterone shots to encourage facial hair, increase muscles and lower their voice, they instead must take shots that increase female hormones right on the other end of the spectrum.

In the US, around 1.4 million adults identify as transgender,[345] but it's estimated only up to five percent of those without children have banked eggs or sperm for the future.[346] [347] This could be partly as people are coming out as transgender or gender nonconforming at earlier ages and stages, when they are less likely to be able to afford fertility preservation treatment on top of other surgical costs, and younger trans people are less likely to have had biological children prior to transitioning.

Additionally, discriminatory definitions in insurance policies mean that trans people, as well as other LGBTQ people, may not meet medical requirements for coverage. Insurance companies often rely on a specific definition of infertility (a man and a woman unable to conceive after having unprotected sex for six to twelve months) to deny coverage to LGBTQ+ people.

DOCTOR INSIGHT: "In my experience, many people planning to undergo gender reassignment don't want to store their eggs. It requires a pregnancy in them, or a surrogate." - Professor Richard Anderson, University of Edinburgh MRC Centre for Reproductive Health

Question 13: Does egg freezing conflict with any of my beliefs?

Ever since the late 1970s, when the world's first "test tube" baby, Louise Brown, was born, there has been something of a tussle over how religions handle reproductive technologies. Attitudes still vary from enthusiastic acceptance to outright opposition. While they don't tend to be over the moon about it, many of the world's major religions tolerate IVF and egg freezing, albeit with certain restrictions. Be aware, though, that that is not the case for the Catholic Church. The Vatican's official position is to reject most forms of fertility treatment (including embryo freezing and the injection of sperm into eggs), with the reasoning being that they are a "substitute" for sex "which alone is truly worthy of responsible procreation." In the Catholic Church's view, a husband and wife should be the only "co-operators with God for giving life to a new person." However, it does actually permit egg freezing. If you do find you need fertility assistance akin to IVF further down the line, some clinics have work-around options that could potentially be possible and are allowed by the church, such as having eggs and sperm transferred to fallopian tubes rather than fertilized in the lab.

DOCTOR INSIGHT: "Religion, and thus, different regulators in different countries, play a crucial role in what is or is not allowed in terms of ART in different countries across the globe. Interestingly, some religions are quite permissive while others are extremely conservative. For example, Catholicism is one of the most strict religions against some treatments, however allows egg freezing. On the other hand, Hinduism, for example, is quite open." - Dr. Juan García Velasco, IVI Madrid, IVI India, IVI GCC

Even where a religion theoretically allows egg freezing, note that there may be particular conditions assigned by religious authorities. For instance, Orthodox Jewish leaders often say that women who freeze their eggs must only use them when they are married and that the procedure must be done under religious supervision. In Islam, which was the first of the major world religion to give assisted reproductive technologies the ok, egg freezing is not "haram" (forbidden). However, the issue is what you do with the eggs later: it is only permissible to use your own eggs, not to donate them, and only married couples are allowed to use IVF. If this might be of concern to you, discuss it with a variety of religious leaders and theologians to make sure you have the benefit of all interpretations and viewpoints.

Broadly, it is a difficult thing to consider the birth of a child "wrong", no matter how she or he was conceived. Many religious people support egg freezing as "pro life" and consider it part of a duty to heal.[348] As well as their objections, bear in mind the Vatican also explicitly says that although assisted reproductive technologies cannot be approved, every child that comes into the world "must in any case be accepted as a living gift of the divine Goodness and must be brought up with love."[349] Even the father of the first "test tube" baby, Louise Brown, who, along with his wife struggled for nine years with infertility before Louise came along, celebrated her birth by telling reporters: "I am not a religious man, but I thank God that I heard our little girl cry for the first time." Her mother, Lesley, said simply: "Louise is, truly, a gift from God."

It's not just religion that might factor into your concerns, but perhaps it's your approach to life. Some women who take considerable care to eat clean, organic foods and keep their bodies away from unnatural things, even avoiding oral birth control, are uncomfortable with the idea of taking injections and are concerned about the potential effects of hormones. While there are no known long-term side effects of injecting yourself, for a short period of time, with higher doses of hormones than are naturally found in your body, some doctors admit that we just can't know the full and subtle long-term impacts of the procedure. If you have any concerns about this, discuss it thoroughly with a doctor and any other expert you value, such as a naturopath, to better inform your decision. In figuring out your philosophy on this, it might be helpful to reflect on the words of Patrick Steptoe, one of the doctors responsible for Louise Brown's birth: "We have merely done what many people try to do in all kinds of medicine — to help nature. We found nature could not put an egg and sperm together, so we did it." He described the procedure as being no more and no less mundanely medical than any other operation, when it comes down to it.

Ultimately, it is for you to make your own informed decision, despite what a specialist, be they a fertility doctor or a religious leader, recommends.

Question 14: What are my other options if I don't freeze my eggs?

Leave it to nature

Regardless of fertility treatment advancements, trying to conceive naturally is the first step for generally healthy people. Only after trying for more than a year (or more than six months if you are over 35 years old) is it considered necessary to consider a consultation with a fertility doctor. After doing the Fertility Forecast exercise, you'll have a better idea of what age you might be likely to be ready to start a family and what your fertility realities are at that age.

That being said, some couples and individuals choose to undergo IVF even if they're not struggling with infertility. According to Dr. Chavkin from HRC Fertility in Los Angeles, "If someone has a genetic condition and they would like their embryo tested for the condition - for instance, if they are a carrier for cystic fibrosis - then they may want to do IVF so that they could do pre-implantation genetic screening (PGS) on the embryo. Or, if they are in their late 30s or early 40s and concerned about the risk of miscarriage or chromosomal abnormalities, they may want to do IVF with their younger eggs, or IVF with their older eggs and test with PGS for chromosomal abnormalities."

In vitro fertilization (IVF)

If you struggle to become pregnant or stay pregnant, a fertility doctor may try a series of fertility treatments, such as medication to stimulate ovulation, with or without intrauterine insemination (IUI), for instance. If these initial interventions don't work, the next step may be IVF treatment. Though sometimes IVF is done using your own cycle ("natural IVF"), generally IVF starts with using hormones to stimulate your ovaries in the same capacity as egg freezing (if you had frozen your eggs you might skip this step and progress to the next after thawing your younger, frozen eggs). If an egg is successfully fertilized in the lab, the embryo can be implanted in your womb. Prior to that, you may wish to do pre-implantation genetic screening to identify an embryo that is chromosomally normal. Note, though, that some people have moral or religious concerns about this kind of testing, which reduces the chance of having a baby with heritable disorders.[350] [351]

IVF comes with a hefty price tag at about $23,747 on average per cycle in the US,[352] and this amount can multiply with the need to go through multiple cycles.[353] [354] Often, the majority of costs of IVF are not covered by insurance plans and people end up paying out of pocket. By age 43, the chance of becoming pregnant through IVF is less than five percent, and by age 45, use of donor eggs is often the only reasonable alternative. The benefit of freezing younger eggs is that, if you do end up needing to use IVF, you are likely to need far fewer cycles to have a baby than if you were using your older eggs, not only saving personal discomfort and potential heartache, but also money.

Use donor eggs

If neither natural conception nor IVF are successful with your own eggs (fresh or frozen), another option is to use another woman's donated eggs. Her eggs would be fertilized with your partner's sperm or donor sperm (in the lab) and then transferred into your womb, or a surrogate's womb. In 2016, more than 24,000 ART cycles were conducted with the use of a donated egg or embryo. This has a higher success rate than non-donor IVF, as donated eggs are usually from women under 35, sometimes under 30 and, as we covered, egg age is the primary barrier to pregnancy in older women, not womb age.[355] While using donor eggs also doesn't guarantee a pregnancy, it offers you the chance to carry a child, albeit one not biologically related to you.

That being said, there have been preliminary studies indicating that, in rare instances, mothers who carry donor eggs may actually still pass on a very small portion of their own DNA (microRNA) to the baby through pregnancy.[356] Some women who use egg donors have taken the news there may be some possibility of a genetic connection through carrying the baby as exciting. It has stirred up interest among those using surrogates to carry their own genetic baby, too, as to the extent of influence the carrier's DNA could have. While the science is interesting and still being researched, doctors stress that the DNA transfer is in reality extremely minimal and very unlikely to have a measurable influence on the genetics of the child.

DOCTOR INSIGHT: "While technically microRNAs from the gestational mother (woman who carries the baby) may pass to the fetal circulation, there is no way any of that DNA is going to medically alter the nuclear DNA, i.e. the genetic makeup of the fetus." - Dr. Carolyn Givens, Pacific Fertility Center, San Francisco

Adopt

People who adopt have no biological tie to their child, but say it can be just as rewarding an experience as biological parenthood. In the US, nearly half a million kids are in foster care[357] and only about 140,000 kids are adopted every year.[358] About 60% of non-step-parent adoptions are from the foster system, where there are plenty of kids in need of good homes. Around a quarter of non-step-parent adoptions are from other countries and 15% are voluntarily relinquished American babies.

The average age of a waiting child is 7.7 years old, but over half of the kids up for adoption are six years old and under.[359] Although only two percent of Americans have adopted, one-third say they have considered it.[360] Parents of adopted children are usually couples in their 30s to mid-40s and single adoptive parents are often women in their 40s.[361]

Of course, the process does come with its challenges. To get more information, visit the Child Welfare Information Gateway, a service of the Children's Bureau, Administration for Children and Families (ACF), which offers in-depth information and resources to assist prospective adoptive parents.

The takeaway:

Now you've considered these questions - some of which are admittedly pretty thought-provoking and tough to answer immediately(!) - the final decision to freeze your eggs is one for you to make along with your doctor's input and advice. Bear in mind that not everyone is considered a good candidate for the egg freezing procedure, which a doctor can only determine after your initial scan, blood test and medical consultation (though second opinions are always advisable), so it's worth going and having these run without delay.

Chapter 5: Setting Expectations

"The pessimist complains about the wind; the optimist expects it to change; the realist adjusts the sails."

— *William Arthur Ward*

While egg freezing and fertility technologies, in general, are advancing year on year, there are some potential eventualities that you should fully absorb before making your decision. Egg freezing isn't part of your everyday life, so let's really level with you for a bit, to try to reduce the chance of any unwelcome surprises:

You might only get a few eggs

It can feel like an incredible disappointment if you get fewer eggs than expected. Women say their first feeling was like their fertility, womanhood, youth and body were somehow not up to scratch. Of course, that's simply not true. Besides the fact that fertility decline is a totally normal, natural and womanly thing, there could be any number of inputs that could be adjusted: your medication type and dose, your lifestyle, even sometimes just month to month variety, that could mean a better result with another cycle. Or maybe another cycle will also yield lower than expected numbers - at that point your doctor can discuss other options with you.

Pre-testing (AMH and AFC and consultation with a fertility doctor) will give you a good indication of your likely expected outcome before you commit to doing a cycle, but you should always consider the possibility the result isn't as predicted. There's a lot out of your direct control. Would you feel short changed if you got fewer eggs than you signed up for? Would you be glad you gave it a shot anyway?

Even when it comes to the things you do control, be aware that this is life, and things can go wrong. For example, we know of one woman who accidentally took the injections in the wrong sequence and ended up with no eggs retrieved as a result. (The good news is, she did another cycle and was satisfied with how many she retrieved that round.)

The best thing to do is to try to calmly manage your expectations beforehand. In a study into the emotional impact of egg freezing, the results showed that women were much more likely to experience regret if they froze ten or fewer eggs, compared with those who had been able to freeze more than ten eggs, so not getting many eggs can be crushing.[362] With all this risk, are the chances you'll get enough eggs to feel satisfied still worth it? For many women, yes. The feeling of *having at least tried* is not to be underestimated. On the whole, 89% of the women in the study above said they were glad they froze their eggs even if they never used them, while 88% said the procedure made them feel as if they had more options for their life.[363] You can't put a price on feeling empowered. And, although money doesn't grow on trees, there may be the option to do another round.

You might need multiple cycles

Depending on your age and the number/quality of eggs retrieved, there's a chance that undergoing multiple cycles would be recommended by your doctor in order to increase your chances of having one healthy baby down the line, especially if you want more than one. And the older you get, the fewer eggs you are likely to retrieve in a single cycle, which is why the average number of cycles increases with each year of age (something to also consider when it comes to cost and deciding at what age to freeze your eggs).

DOCTOR PERSPECTIVE: "My average patient going through egg freezing is over 30 years old. I encourage freezing enough eggs to give women at least two kids from their frozen eggs. So it isn't unusual for my patients to do two or even three cycles." - Dr. Aimee Eyvazzadeh, Private Practice Physician, San Ramon

Your eggs could get damaged or destroyed

While storage facility failures are incredibly rare, they do happen. Cryopreservation facilities are not immune from human error, accidents, destructive weather or natural disasters. There could also be human errors in the laboratory when handling, freezing or thawing your eggs. There are ways to reduce your risk of this happening. First and foremost, select a high quality clinic and ask the right questions about their storage facility (see the list of questions provided in Chapter 6, "Picking the Clinic"). Some people even recommend storing your eggs in separate facilities in order to quite literally avoid putting all your eggs in one basket. However, this too comes with a very small risk that your eggs will be damaged in transport and you might have to pay double the storage fees. You could always ask the clinic to split your eggs into more than one storage tank, instead. As your eggs are human tissue utterly unique to you, there is no way to insure against their potential loss.

Egg freezing can be an emotional process

For many women, egg freezing marks a specific time in life. The very decision itself can trigger introspection and lead you to evaluate life events or choices, as well as trying to piece together what the future may hold. Then, when it comes to the hormone injections, you could experience a heightened version of whatever emotions you tend to feel during PMS - the intensity and precise nature of the effect are different for everyone.

For us, the process certainly came with its highs and lows, be they crying at commercials (Brittany) or getting way too into Spotify (Catherine). It's hard to boil it down to just one emotion as egg freezing can invoke a fuzz of different feelings in one day, from excited to isolated to empowered to pensive and back again. But in the end, we both felt after we'd done it we could breathe a little easier, with a bit of weight off our shoulders. The clock was ticking a little less insistently.

It's best to plan for the worst and hope for the best. A lot of women carry on working and socializing as normal for the majority of the cycle. But it doesn't hurt to stock up on magazines and snacks just in case. (We'll look at the emotional side of things in more detail in Part Three.)

Chapter 6: Picking the Clinic

"It does not take much strength to do things, but it requires a great deal of strength to decide what to do."

— *Elbert Hubbard*

There are around 500 fertility clinics in the US and more are cropping up every year (meaning there's plenty to choose from!).[364] Reproductive medicine is a very competitive specialty for doctors, but despite this, not all clinics and doctors are created equal. The fertility industry is a fast-growing market; labs are easy to start and surprisingly loosely regulated,[365] so it's essential to do your homework and make sure you're trusting your eggs to the best possible team.

In lieu of formal regulation, most likely due to political reasons, there's instead a system of "self-regulation" via industry bodies like the ASRM and SART, which is just something to be aware of when you're doing your due diligence and picking a clinic. If there's one thing you draw from this section, it's that it is vital that you properly vet your potential clinic and only go ahead with a clinician you are comfortable with and who makes sure to counsel you clearly, fairly and openly. Knowing the right questions to ask is important not only for your safety but because the experience of the staff and the quality of the lab can have a tangible impact on the success of your procedure. The step-by-step guide below is designed to make it easy for you to ask all the relevant questions to pick your clinic:

Step 1: Get recommendations from trusted sources

When it comes to picking a clinic, it can be hard to know where to begin. A good place to start is by asking your gynecologist if she or he has recommendations for you. You can assume their recommendations will be based on success or feedback from their other patients, whether it's for egg freezing or other fertility treatments.

If you're open to it, it's also worth asking your friends and friends-of-friends to see if they had a clinic or doctor that they'd recommend either for egg freezing or other fertility treatments like IVF. You can also check out the ELANZA fertility doctor directory where you'll get a feel for each doctor's personality and unique approach to patient care. Find it here: www.elanzawellness.com/fertilitydoctors

"Even before I was sure I wanted to freeze my eggs, I wanted to get some of the tests done and talk to a fertility doctor about my options. I found a few websites with patient reviews about various clinics but it just wasn't enough. So I decided to send out a group message to a few of my close friends to see if they know of anyone that had undergone fertility treatment and if they'd be willing to chat about their clinic experience. I was astounded how many of them had their own experiences to share and how open and willing they were to talk about it! I was able to find a fantastic doctor and my friends were so supportive all the way through." - Bryana, 36

"I've had the same gynecologist for years. When I mentioned to her that I was thinking about freezing my eggs, she put me in touch with a clinic that her other patients really loved. She knows me and my health history so it made the whole process really easy to navigate." Cherise, 37

Are you interested in freezing your eggs overseas?

While the cost savings of going overseas can be great, and open up egg freezing to some women who might not otherwise be able to afford it (and can even be a lovely getaway!), there are quite a few important things to take into account before considering traveling overseas for egg freezing:

- **The country itself** - Not all countries' medical, legal and political systems are robust and reliable. It's reported that of the estimated 103 countries around the globe with fertility centers, 42 operate with legislative oversight, 26 with voluntary guidelines, and 35 operate with neither (the US falls into the "voluntary" category). Check which laws, regulations and guidelines are in place for the country you're traveling to and have that form part of your decision making process.[366]

- **Clinic -** Using a clinic overseas obviously makes it harder to swing by to check it out, but gather as many reviews as possible, make sure to video consult with your doctor and check in with the country's fertility industry regulator about the reputation and statistics for the clinic. The same important questions apply as in the US - qualifications, clinic standards and storage security / power backups, but also ask if they regularly have overseas patients and if there is a system to manage them, as this would likely streamline your experience.

- **Price** - Although treatment costs may be substantially lower, flights, transportation, accommodation, insurance and other travel costs must be properly factored in. Even then, the total cost can be far less than in the US. [367] [368] [369]

- **Insurance** - Regular travel insurance will not cover problems arising from the procedure. In some cases, even claims that have nothing to do with the procedure will not be covered if the trip is taken for medical tourism purposes. However, specialist medical travel insurance is available for people traveling specifically for surgery, usually at a reasonable cost.

- **If something goes wrong** - In the very small chance that anything goes medically wrong, consider if you would be comfortable being far from home and potentially alone. Of course, your medical travel insurance should cover any additional hospital stay and treatment, but consider every scenario. Most European countries practicing non-medical freezing do so in the context of the absence of a specific law governing it, for instance.[370] Consider also that many countries have far fewer clear-cut paths for legal recourse if there is gross incompetence or medical negligence - it is often harder to prove than it is in the US legal system. Thankfully, in egg freezing procedures these instances are rare.

- **Using your eggs** - By default, your eggs will be frozen and stored in the country in which you have the procedure. For some women, this makes sense because if you end up choosing to use your frozen eggs, you might want to return for the IVF procedure as you are likely to reap the same cost benefits. It should be noted that some countries such as the UK currently have a time limit on how long eggs can be stored and others do not have sperm banks, for instance, Australia.

- **Transporting your eggs** - If you'd rather have your eggs stored in your home country, you can arrange to have them sent via specialist airmail courier to the storage facility of your choice. This can cost from several hundred dollars to more than $1,000 and involve some administration. Transporting eggs is known to be safe (many US clinics transport eggs to off-site storage facilities), but of course, any additional movement increases risks. Most doctors would advise leaving them in place.

- **Timing** - While you can take the contraceptive pill to time your cycle and plan your travel, the ovarian stimulation cycle isn't a fixed length. For most women, the stimulation cycle will last for 8-12 days but can reach up to 14, not including recovery time. It is possible to fly 24 hours after your procedure, but without knowing how you might feel or in the rare event that there are any complications, you might consider adding on a few days post-procedure to allow time for a full recovery. Seeing as this is a significant amount of time to be away, some women arrange to do the initial injections and monitoring appointments at home, which can cut down on timing. Make sure to discuss this with your doctor beforehand as there may be logistical and financial implications.

- **Language/culture shock** - Check that the clinic staff speaks English and that all documentation will be available translated. Perhaps for you travel will be a relaxing experience, away from day-to-day pressures. But if you rarely travel, going overseas for treatment may be a stressful experience, particularly in countries where there are substantial cultural differences.

- **Admin** - Traveling overseas for treatment can increase the administrative burden of the experience. There are a number of "fertili-travel" companies focused on egg freezing and wellness vacations, or even agents who specialize in helping with clinic selection, travel logistics and medication/appointment coordination while you're there. It's a fast-growing space so check our website to learn more about your options and get some information on the ones we've checked out.

- **Support** - If you are traveling overseas, consider your support systems. Friends and family could check in with you over the phone, but with some women reporting feeling lonely and isolated during the process, it might be worth traveling with a companion.

Step 2: Send questions to clinics to understand quality and costs

Unfortunately, it would basically take a degree in embryology to determine the actual quality of a clinic and lab. While clinics publish success rate statistics for other treatments like IVF, often the historical data just isn't available for planned egg freezing because it's a newer treatment. The other challenge is that the word "success" is a much less tangible concept for egg freezing. In IVF cycles, "success" means a baby born. But for egg freezing, retrieving five eggs for one woman aged 37 with a complex medical history could be considered a great result. Getting, say, fifteen eggs from a younger, healthy woman could be an equivalent win. And without a way to measure the quality of those eggs without fertilizing them, there's actually no way to accurately predict the "success" of the eggs retrieved. However, there is a considerable overlap in the clinical processes used in IVF and for egg freezing, which is why a clinic's IVF success rate can be used as a proxy for their general expertise. However, this doesn't necessarily account for a lab's ability to properly freeze and thaw eggs, which is, as you might imagine, a very important aspect of egg freezing.

This is also a good time to get the full picture on costs.

To help you streamline this process, we've compiled a list of questions for you to send to clinics that address factors like accreditation, skills, experience, success rates as well as a breakdown of costs. You can find a free downloadable template with all the questions and answers to look for at www.ELANZAwellness.com.

Doctor and clinic experience

- Are all of your fertility doctors board certified and members of professional bodies like the American Society for Reproductive Medicine and / or the Society of Reproductive Endocrinologists?

- How many years have you been offering egg freezing? How many egg freezing cycles do you conduct per year?

- Is your clinic open 7 days a week?

- Is your clinic open 365 days a year?

- Who does the monitoring during stimulation? Will I see a doctor vs. a nurse practitioner or an ultrasound tech?

- How often will I see my doctor during the process?

- Will I have a nurse advocate or a single point of contact assigned to me for the duration of the process?

Clinic success rates

- Of the women that have frozen their eggs, how many have come back to use them at your facility? And how many resulted in live births?

- What is your "oocyte (egg) cryosurvival rate?"

- Which method of freezing do you use? I.e. slow freezing or vitrification

- What percentage of fertilized eggs survive to day 5?

- Do you culture your embryos beyond day 6 when creating embryos from frozen eggs?

Storage facility quality

- Where will my eggs be stored?

- What monitoring systems do you have in place for the nitrogen tanks?

- What are your backup procedures in case of a power failure or natural disaster (e.g. earthquake)?

- Can I transport my eggs to another fertility clinic to use or store?

Initial costs

- What is the initial consultation fee and what does it cover?

Step 3: Set up initial conversations/consultations with your top 2-3 clinics

These can be introductory chats with a look around the clinic or full consultations with the doctors (according to your budget, as most will charge for a clinical consultation). Many clinics now offer egg freezing Q&A events and webcasts led by a doctor or nurse who can guide you through their clinic's approach and can answer any of the questions you may have. This is a great (free!) way to start gathering more detailed knowledge about the procedure and the differences between clinics.

Once you get your basic questions answered, you'll need to setup a private consultation with a clinic or two. Clinics usually charge for this, which will cost you between $150 and $400. The consultation will usually involve: doctor consultation (included); transvaginal ultrasound (included); blood work (charged separately). You can do just one of these at the clinic you have chosen, or you might prefer to compare two or three, depending on your budget. Note that some insurance plans may cover this consultation. Some clinics may have appointment waiting lists of a few months, so try to do this as soon as possible before the time you think you want to freeze your eggs. In case there is a long waiting period, you can get a head start on optimizing your eggs with the lifestyle modifications outlined in Part Two of this guide.

Step 4: Breakdown the costs for each clinic

Oftentimes you will meet with a clinic's financial consultant on the same day as your initial doctor consultation. They'll walk you through all the costs as well as any financing options they might have available. Some clinics will provide you with a lump sum, others a break-down. To avoid any hidden costs, make sure to ask for a breakdown of all the fees. Some clinics offer financing, such as paying for a certain number of eggs frozen, regardless of the number of cycles, or paying a fixed, reduced fee for multiple cycles. Ask what deals a clinic can offer you. We've broken down what the costs might be and what you might expect to pay for them. Keep in mind that these costs can vary greatly by clinic, mostly influenced by where they're located.

Cost 2 - Diagnostic tests:

Blood tests such as AMH will help inform your doctor about how well you might respond to treatment. These are almost always charged separately.
Estimated cost: $175 - $700, depending on tests required.

Cost 3 - Egg freezing cycle:

This is the core of what the fertility clinic will charge you. This usually includes the 3-6 scans conducted at the clinic during the stimulation phase to see how your follicles are progressing, the cost of the 15-30-minute retrieval surgery, and the lab processing fees for freezing the eggs.
Estimated cost: +/- $7,000. Some clinics will offer a discount on subsequent cycles, if they are merited.

Cost 4 - Medication:

This covers the cost of the hormone injections required to stimulate and manage your ovaries over the course of stimulation phase. This is very seldom included in the clinic's pricing. The doctor will only decide which medications and in what dosage you need once he or she sees how your follicles are progressing. Some women simply require more than others, which is why the costs can vary. Your doctor might be able to give you an estimate on how much medication you'll need in order to anticipate cost, but once your doctor creates your stimulation protocol, you will need to purchase your medication directly from a pharmacy.

Estimated cost: $2,500 - $6,500 per cycle.

Cost 5 - Storage:

This is an annual cost to keep your eggs frozen in a specialized facility. This is a hidden cost that can really add up, especially if you plan on storing them for a while. Many clinics have their own storage facilities on site or nearby and will often include the first year free as part of the total treatment cost. But you also have the option of storing them elsewhere. For example, there are some storage facilities that are located in super secure earthquake free zones and can often offer more competitive rates. The one downside of this is the very small risk that something could happen to them in transit (think odds of a plane crash).

Estimated cost: $450 to $1,100 per year.

Step 4: Prepare for your consultation by getting screening tests beforehand

When setting up the appointment, ask if there are specific tests or medical history information you can have prepared before the consultation. Some tests are used to measure your fertility potential and others are general health safeguards that are legally required before you can proceed with treatment. When it comes to the general health screenings, you can expect to need some or all of the following: blood type and screen, complete blood count (CBC), thyroid stimulating hormone (TSH), a complete sexually transmitted infection (STI) screening, a Pap smear, and a mammogram report (only if you are 40+). Most of these tests can either be facilitated by your gynecologist and primary care physician. If you've had any of these tests conducted in the last year, just confirm with the clinic because you might not need to take them again. If you're not able to get the requested tests in time, some clinics will be able to do some of the tests at the time of your consultation, and as long as you get them done before the cycle begins it shouldn't be a huge problem. But you'll make much more out of your consultation if your doctor has all your information beforehand. In some countries with different care systems, such as the UK, you may go to a fertility clinic straight off the bat for your consultation, tests, monitoring and procedure, without needing to visit your GP first. If you prefer, you can chat to your GP to ask for recommendations or a referral, though.

In addition to your general health screenings, most doctors will also request that you get a blood test to measure your anti-Mullerian hormone (AMH) levels. This is one of the two main tests used by doctors to understand how many eggs you may still have left in your ovaries, which forms part of what is often referred to as your "ovarian reserve" and can also inform doctors on the dosage of medication to prescribe you over the stimulation cycle.

Put simply, AMH is a hormone emitted by the immature follicles resting inside your ovaries. The more resting follicles you have, the higher your AMH levels, and vice versa. Seeing as your follicle count decreases with age, you can expect that your level of AMH will decline accordingly. But for some people, this rate of decline comes sooner than later. So what is considered a good AMH level for egg freezing? According to our Expert Panelist, Dr. Westphal, "There is some variation in the data. I would say 1-3.5 is normal, 3.5-5 is borderline high and over 5 is high (and may be associated with PCOS)." It should also be noted that AMH testing is not a perfect science. Your AMH levels may be affected by factors such as oral contraceptives and smoking. And, this test only hints at the quantity of eggs you have left, which ignores an equally important factor, the quality. Regardless of its limitations, it will help your doctor advise on whether egg freezing is a good option for you.

If you aren't able to get your AMH levels tested beforehand, the clinic can most likely take a blood sample during your consultation. Just make sure to bring copies of your test results or have them emailed to the fertility clinics before your consultation.

What about at-home fertility tests?

You may have noticed a few companies popping up that offer at-home fertility tests. We're all for being proactive about your fertility and taking steps to do so, and these tests can be a good way to start getting informed. However, just remember not to read too much into your results without trained eyes interpreting them: it's easy for the results to get taken out of context. Fertility doctors are specifically trained to utilize a variety of tests and medical history to best interpret the results.

Although AMH hormone tests are good for measuring, well, your AMH levels, researchers have found there's little correlation between these egg store test scores and your chances of actually getting pregnant. In a study of women who were trying to get pregnant naturally, low AMH levels indicating diminished ovarian reserve were not associated with infertility. Basically, ovarian reserve tests are a good measure of how many eggs you have left (and could be a good indication of how you might respond to ovarian stimulation in an egg freezing cycle), but that alone doesn't predict your reproductive potential, or, to put it another way, your fertility.

The takeaway here is to be careful not to come to any conclusions based on the results of one of these tests alone. Always seek a full consultation with a fertility specialist doctor. And if you are going to use a test, doctors rate the "finger prick" blood tests far more highly than the pee sticks.

"I did an AMH test and the results came back suggesting that I was completely infertile at age 34! While I wasn't ready for kids at that moment, I knew I wanted them one day and I was totally crushed. Because I was 'infertile' I decided to be a little more liberal in the bedroom with a guy I was very casually seeing. And then, literally the next month I was pregnant. I was totally unprepared for a child, emotionally or practically, but I felt like it could be my only chance. I might be an extreme case, but one little stick changed the entire course of my life." - Malia, 36

Step 5: Assess the clinics and consult with the doctors

As you narrow down your options, having an in-person consultation at one or more clinics is important for a few reasons. First, this is your chance to get your full fertility assessment from the doctor, including any additional tests as well as answers to any questions you might have about how they operate and what kind of outcome you might expect. But second, it's an opportunity to get a feel for the clinic and its style. It's important that you feel both comfortable and confident in a clinic's surroundings - you'll be spending a decent amount of time there. Do you feel like the staff is helpful, organized, and communicative? Do they seem focused on personalized care? How efficiently was the appointment booking process?

In addition to the screening tests already mentioned, most doctors will want to conduct an ultrasound to determine something called your antral follicle count (AFC). This, combined with the results from your anti-Mullerian hormone (AMH) test are considered the best means in which to understand your fertility.[371] [372] To get this measurement, the doctor or an ultrasound technician will take a look at your ovaries. This could be a transabdominal ultrasound (like the ones you've probably seen used on pregnant women in movies), but most often they will use a "transvaginal" ultrasound (this is effectively a wand-like object covered in a condom and lubrication, which is inserted into your vagina). You might feel a pressure sensation but it's not generally painful. While the doctor or technician moves the wand around to get a good look at both your ovaries, she or he is looking to measure the quantity and size of your follicles (i.e. the fluid-filled sacs that contain your eggs).

How many antral follicles are considered "normal?" Doctors on our expert panel say that this number can fluctuate from zero to 30 for a woman the same age but for the purposes of egg freezing, they like to see an AFC of >10. Keep in mind that this only tells part of the story behind your fertility potential.

DOCTOR INSIGHT: "Antral follicle counts can vary from provider to provider, as there is no real accepted consensus on how small is too small to count as an antral follicle. Also, the antral follicles present in an ovary at any one moment in time are always in transition. Some are just coming into the antral pool and some are on their way to the fate of almost all antral follicles and eggs within: reabsorption by the body. We cannot tell the difference. This is why I tell my patients that I do the count as a guideline to choose the dose of stimulation medication for them and to help to set a 'ballpark' estimation on the final number of eggs we might obtain from a subsequent egg freezing cycle." - Dr. Carolyn Givens, Pacific Fertility Center, San Francisco

Once you've reviewed the tests with your doctor, he or she will be able to advise on whether or not egg freezing is right for you. This is also your chance to ask many of the questions specific to your own fertility such as the potential risks from the procedure, and what kind of outcome you can expect. For example: How many cycles do you think I will need? Am I at a high risk for Ovarian Hyperstimulation Syndrome (OHSS)? Are there any other risks that are specific to me?

While you're with the doctor, don't feel shy about asking any and all questions about the process and the procedure that you might be unclear about. This is especially important in the clinic selection phase because the approach, perspective and process can differ, sometimes dramatically, from doctor-to-doctor. Having a doctor that you resonate with could make all the difference.

If you don't have a good experience or if you want a second opinion, don't stop there. Even if it means setting up additional consultations at a different clinics, it will be worth it to know you're freezing your eggs with a team who show the right care, expertise, experience and professionalism.

Step 6: Pick the winner

Once you've checked out your shortlist options, it's time to weigh up your options and - if you've decided to go ahead with at least the consultation - pull the trigger! There's really no time like the present...

EXPERT INSIGHT: "Choosing the right clinic is important so you feel comfortable regardless if it is a clinic far away or near your home base. Choosing the right clinic is a very personal choice and each person needs to decide what is important to them. I personally went to three different fertility clinics. I chose a different fertility center each cycle of my freezes so as to not put all my eggs in one basket. I had a great experience each time and with each group. Trusting your medical team is key to having a good experience. Being comfortable to ask questions and be able to reach medical staff on demand can help any uncertainties." - Valerie Landis, Fertility Patient Advocate

Decision time: food for thought

There's plenty to muse over - from your own personal cost benefit analysis, to which clinic, to when the right time in your busy life might present itself...this isn't a decision that should be rushed, for sure.

And yet, we wouldn't be presenting the full reality of the situation if we didn't reemphasize that age is the most important factor at play. Fertility doctors we speak to often despair that the vast majority of women they see for egg freezing don't come to them until their late thirties. It's not that it's a pointless exercise then, far from it. It's just, from their clinical perspective, it would give you more chance of a better outcome in the long term if you freeze younger eggs.

The point is, if after careful consideration you think you do want to egg freeze, don't wait for some ideal moment: that moment may never come. Sometimes, you have to take what you want while it's there for the taking. You will never be younger than you are today.

Part one summary

- Age-related fertility decline results from several factors: decreasing egg count, reduced ovarian responsiveness to hormones, general health declining with age and - most critically - the quality of your eggs.[373]

- Egg freezing is considered a safe and effective tool to protect your fertility potential, though there are no guarantees.

- There is no exact right time to freeze. The average age of women freezing is 36 years old. Most doctors recommend freezing before age 37. Over age 45, it is not recommended. After completing various screening tests (namely your AMH and AFC) you and your doctor can discuss whether or not you are a candidate for egg freezing.

- The process is generally painless. The injections are a bit intimidating but not necessarily painful. They hormones can give you PMS-like symptoms, especially as you approach your retrieval date. The procedure itself should be painless (thanks to anesthesia). Recovery on the day of retrieval can be uncomfortable but most women are back at work the next day.

- The likelihood that one cycle of egg freezing will result in a future baby is dependent upon (1) your age at the time of freezing and (2) how many eggs were frozen.

- Egg freezing can work because it's the age of your eggs that matter, not the age of your womb, if you decide to use them.

- You would only need to use your frozen eggs if you cannot conceive naturally. If you do decide to use them, you would have them thawed, fertilized with sperm (in a petri dish) and have the resulting embryo implanted into your womb, in the hopes it would result in a successful pregnancy.

- Egg freezing is not guaranteed. You might only get a few eggs from a cycle. You might need multiple cycles to retrieve more eggs. Your eggs could get damaged.

- Your lifestyle choices can have an effect on the quality and quantity of eggs retrieved.

- A doctor's experience and the quality of the lab can affect your outcome. Ask plenty of questions when finding the right clinic for you.

PART TWO: PREPARING YOUR EGGS FOR FREEZING

Get Fertility Fit™ three to four months before the stimulation cycle begins

"Do something today that your future self will thank you for."

– Anonymous

So, if you've decided to freeze your eggs: doesn't it feel good to have chosen a course of action?! So now, sit back and settle in for the ride. Let the preparations commence!

You've seen in Part One that lifestyle changes *can* influence fertility: in this section we get to the cool bit, what exactly those changes are. Here's your opportunity to refine your lifestyle in ways that could enhance the quality of your eggs, both for your upcoming egg freezing cycle and beyond.

> *DOCTOR INSIGHT: "As a clinician, I've seen plenty of women who have had undesirable results from their first egg retrieval, and then take three months to focus on specific health and lifestyle modifications before going back for another cycle. Almost every single time, the woman gets more egg retrieved and the embryos are better quality." - Dr. Jenn Shulman, Jennifer Shulman Acupuncture, New York and Los Angeles*

Why make lifestyle changes: are they really worth the effort?

In a word, yes. Consider this an opportunity for a better outcome, a better experience, and better long term reproductive health. Lifestyle changes work. Hundreds of studies show, for instance, that specific dietary patterns translate to better fertility treatment outcomes, such as higher quality eggs, higher number of eggs retrieved,[374] increased pregnancy rates,[375] [376] and lower risks of miscarriage.[377]

There's a vast body of research out there, so we've whittled it down to the lifestyle factors that could enhance your egg freezing outcome, without causing you harm, that you might practically and realistically be able to make.

"Up until recently, I spent my entire life trying NOT to get pregnant. So when I decided to freeze my eggs I had to make a major mental shift. And I quickly realized that I didn't know anything about fertility. An online search provided disappointing results that fell into one of two categories: indecipherable medical journals and amateur health bloggers raving about turmeric." - Sharman, 33

"When I froze my eggs I didn't realize there were things I could do to prep my body beforehand. I didn't make any lifestyle changes and I really wish I had. Even without knowing exactly how big of a difference it would have made, I feel like I missed out on potential benefits." - Shannon, 35

Ultimately, with the price of egg freezing, don't you want to know you did everything you could to get the best result? The efforts you make to refine your lifestyle will help you prepare your eggs in the best way possible for your treatment cycle. What could feel better than knowing you've given yourself the best shot?

How do I know they'll work?

It's said that a lie gets halfway around the world before the truth has a chance to get its pants on - and that's certainly true when it comes to many of the ludicrous fertility fixes you'll find in certain corners of the internet. We've cut out the click bait that add up to nothing more than wasted time, energy and money. Instead, we've stuck with the science. This means clear, practical advice drawn from studies on how you might feel, what to eat, what to cut out, which supplements are worth the money and which lifestyle choices, changes and tweaks are proven to help your body produce its best quality eggs. We think it's great to keep an open mind when it comes to health and lifestyle, but, equally, who wants to spend their evenings gulping down a rancid herbal concoction or wafting a jade egg around their lady parts if there's no data to say that will do anything at all? Time, for us all, is precious. And our fertility even more so.

The lifestyle changes we discuss here are "evidence based." What we mean by that is that you can trust that they are rooted in results from scientific studies and that our Expert Panel think they are either proven beyond doubt, or are at the very least credible and scientifically plausible. High quality, unbiased, relevant and trustworthy evidence is not that easy to come by in general. But, wherever possible, the data we cite is the current best empirical evidence from rigorously evaluated studies, including randomized controlled trials which have shown statistically significant outcomes, plus other recognized methodologies such as descriptive and qualitative research and case studies.

Because there is a real lack of specific studies to date on healthy women freezing their eggs, we have drawn - as doctors do - on the solid and widespread research that has been done on women who are having related treatments, such as IVF, or women who are facing reproductive health problems in general. Incidentally, where we cite non-human studies you'll see they're often on mice. That's because mouse eggs and embryos are routinely used for research and quality control for assisted reproductive technologies, thanks to the difficulties running controlled studies in women and, also, a key skill mice possess: reproducing at lightning speed!

How long should my Fertility Fit™ program be?

Ideally, 90 days. Think of it as a three-month Fertility Fit™ bootcamp for your ovaries that runs in tandem with your doctor's advice and care. This time frame aligns with that three month "rapid growth" window that you might remember from Part One.

If three months isn't realistic for your situation (if you've already got the procedure booked, or your doctor advises doing the procedure as soon as possible, for instance if you're awaiting chemotherapy and every second counts), then work with the time you have. The benefits could still help your outcome. Oh, and if we've said it once we've said it a thousand times: adopting many of these habits will be good for your long-term reproductive health! So, every positive step matters.

But, bear in mind there are a few particular things that might be worth getting in check before you get started...

Top two pivotal lifestyle changes: smoking and weight

If you're a cigarette smoker

One of the most colossal changes you can make for your short and long-term fertility is to quit smoking.[378] Doctors have told us that the ovaries of women who smoke can look more like those of women up to five years older. The scientific evidence is also clear. Smoking can reduce your overall fertility by 60%.[379] It's linked with everything from irregular periods[380] to a diminished ovarian reserve,[381] which makes sense why smokers are more likely to go through menopause one to four years earlier than women who don't.[382] [383] [384] [385] Every year of smoking has been shown to increase the risk of unsuccessful IVF by up to nine percent[386] and the risk of miscarriage increases by one percent per cigarette smoked per day.[387]

In ovarian stimulation cycles, smokers' egg quality appears to be lower than that of non-smokers. This is evidenced by the fact that smokers undergoing IVF have more canceled cycles (usually due to poor egg development), lower implantation rates and more cycles with failed fertilization compared to non-smokers.[388] [389] [390] [391] [392] [393] This is also supported by research showing that women who smoke are more likely to conceive a chromosomally unhealthy pregnancy (such as a pregnancy affected by Down syndrome) than non-smoking mothers.[394] One culprit is a group of chemicals called polycyclic aromatic hydrocarbons (PAHs) found in cigarette smoke are known to accelerate the destruction of your eggs by causing DNA damage to the ovarian follicles, where the eggs normally develop to maturity.[395] [396]

It's unclear how much of the damage is reversible but one large study showed that when women stopped smoking, the risk of earlier menopause decreased.[397] What is clear is that the sooner you quit, the better it is for your fertility.

DOCTOR INSIGHT: "Smoking is one of the worst things for egg quality. Stop sucking on the egg killers is what I tell my patients. Nicotine levels can literally be measured in a smoking woman's ovaries!" - Dr. Aimee Eyvazzadeh, Private Practice Physician, San Ramon

What about electronic cigarettes, vaping, or twisps?

There's no doubt that without the thousands of carcinogens found in cigarette smoke (e.g. lead, arsenic, hydrogen cyanide, formaldehyde, and uranium(!?), to name a few), e-cigarettes are *less* bad than cigarettes. On the other hand, the aerosols produced by e-cigs can contain nicotine, flavorings, and a variety of other chemicals, some of which are known to be toxic.[398] At this moment, the specific short and long-term effects on fertility are not known, but it's still concerning enough for at least 16 authorities in the UK to introduce a policy refusing couples access to state-sponsored IVF treatment if they use e-cigarettes or nicotine patches![399]

Does secondhand smoke matter?

Signs point to yes. While the evidence is limited, one study found that patients exposed to secondhand smoke ("passive smokers") had the same lower pregnancy rates as smokers, though this could be due to effects on the womb, rather than egg quality.[400] Further evidence comes from a study in which 84% of women who reported themselves as nonsmokers with smoking partners had detectable levels of cotinine (a major metabolite of nicotine that can have a negative impact on fertilization rates[401]) in the follicular fluid surrounding their eggs upon retrieval during IVF.[402] If you often find yourself in the company of smokers, try asking them to smoke outdoors, avoiding enclosed spaces where you're more likely to get secondhand exposure. Your doctor can suggest a range of resources and support to help you quit smoking in a manageable way.

If you have weight issues

If you have significant struggles with your weight (on the very top or the lowest side of the scale) you may want to take longer to make some changes before your egg freezing cycle, as all these things are established fertility foes. It's important not to try to make drastic lifestyle changes overnight, as this can put your body under a great deal of stress. For example, if you are severely overweight or underweight, a 20% rapid gain or loss in the opposite direction could cause menstrual irregularities and cause a hormonal imbalance.[403] Taking your time to make healthy and steady lifestyle changes that are sustainable over time is by far your best strategy.

If you're on the heavier side

If you are above average weight, you should consider losing some body fat prior to your egg freezing cycle, to optimize your outcome. We are big supporters of body positivity, so this is not about body shaming or saying we've all got to look one uniform way *at all*. Culturally, artistically and romantically, there's no right or wrong. However, scientifically, we're on different ground. Science is an out-and-out body shamer, and it is pointing the finger and saying that, in general, women who are heavier than a body mass index (BMI) of 25 have more fertility issues. By heavier, doctors usually use the terms "overweight" (classified as a BMI of 25–29.9) and "obese" (BMI of 30 and above.) There are plenty of free online BMI measurement tools that can help see if you fall into a fertility-friendly bodyweight.

BMI is a notoriously tricky thing, of course. That's why spreadsheets and data tables are great on the one hand, but on the other hand they really have their limits. They're a little...reductive. When you just look at a number, there's no context and no subtlety. We all know that you can be bigger or wear a plus size and still be perfectly healthy, especially if you're eating great things and working out. So, when scientists say the optimal weight for fertility that they've identified is a body mass index (BMI) of 20-25, you've of course got to use some intelligent judgment. If you're an athlete, or you have always just been super strong, or you know you live a healthy lifestyle but still that number comes out weird, then this probably won't be a real concern - discuss it with your doctor. However, if you know your diet and exercise choices aren't ideal and you're carrying more body fat than lean muscle, this is the time to get activated.

BMI Formula

703 x weight (lbs)

height (in)²

So what are the fertility problems? Research suggests that overweight and obese women are much more likely to experience anovulation, menstrual disorders,[404] infertility, difficulties in assisted reproduction, miscarriage, and adverse pregnancy outcomes.[405] [406] [407] [408] [409] [410] Even with the help of hormones used in the egg freezing process, most studies show that obese women going through IVF tend to have fewer eggs retrieved, fewer mature eggs, and poorer egg quality compared to women who are not overweight or obese.[411] [412] [413] [414] [415] [416] [417] [418] [419] [420] [421] In fact, being obese is directly considered a risk factor for infertility.[422] [423]

One culprit for these infertility issues is rooted in the fact that your fat cells produce estrogen in addition to the estrogen already being produced in your ovaries. As such, the more fat cells you have, the more your body creates unnecessary amounts of estrogen. This excess estrogen has a domino effect on other hormones, throwing them all out of balance, causing reproductive issues such as irregular ovulation.[424]

Being overweight also influences other factors that are problematic for reproduction, including stress, lack of sleep, insulin resistance, oxidative stress and more, which we'll cover in the following chapters. For those with a more substantial percentage of weight to lose in order to get to a BMI below 25, the good news is that even a five percent reduction in weight has been shown to improve fertility.[425] [426] [427] This can also help lower your risk of complications while under anesthesia.[428] It's better to aim for a smaller, steadier weight loss, even if you don't immediately move into this "optimal" BMI range. It's not just about egg freezing - the healthy lifestyle changes that lead to weight loss will have an immediate impact on long-term fertility and your overall well being – meaning you don't have to cross the finish line into this BMI range before seeing improvements in egg quantity and quality.

This isn't about declaring war on your fat cells or sending you into a struggle against your own body. The intention here is not weight loss in and of itself, or weight loss to fit a cultural condition of how you "should" look in clothes. This is fat loss and weight loss as side effects of lifestyle changes that may improve your fertility. The super simple principles in the "Eating for Egg Health" chapter are there to help you transition into a new kind of healthy balance, to plan for your future.

If you're on the slimmer side

People kind of laugh at the term "skinny shaming" as if it doesn't exist and it's not a real and hurtful form of body policing. Well, the optimal fertility scale is back, and it's running its judgy eye over slimmer women, too. That's to say, the data suggests that having a BMI of 20 or less also comes with a higher risk of infertility.[429] [430]

If your BMI is under 20 you are more likely to have an ovulatory disorder,[431] a higher risk of miscarriage,[432] ovarian dysfunction[433] and pregnancy issues such as preterm birth.[434] This happens in part because key sex hormones like estrogen are produced and stored in fat cells. So, just as heavier women produce *excess* estrogen, skinnier women, who have less of what's been coined "sex fat" (tissue where sex hormones are stored) can have lower estrogen levels.[435]

Being very slim can also inhibit the production of other key fertility hormones such as leptin, which is thought to give ovaries the green light to function.[436] This is most likely because leptin plays a role in the regulation of energy balance (how many calories you eat, burn and store as fat) and is produced and stored in fat cells. So, when fat cells are in short supply, leptin signals to your body that the conditions are inadequate for reproduction.[437]

Why would your body demand some body fat in order to prepare itself for reproduction? Well, in part because pregnancy and breastfeeding each have high energy costs and place extra daily caloric demands on the body.[438] [439] So when calories are in short supply or you don't have any spare body fat, it makes sense that your body prioritizes its day-to-day living-and-breathing functions over reproductive ones, knowing that an even bigger energy demand could be the result of getting pregnant.

Just as for women who come out on the heavier end of BMI measurements, these indices can be a tricky thing to navigate as some women are naturally very slender, have little body fat or struggle to gain weight. However, if you have low body fat due to a restrictive diet or excessive exercise (more on that later), that could be a red flag for impaired fertility. Although a BMI of over 20 is considered *optimal* for fertility - the Goldilocks zone - your doctor would probably only raise the topic with you if your BMI is under 18, as that's considered a rough tipping point for potential fertility issues.

EXPERT INSIGHT: "If you have a history of eating disorders, you should be open and honest with your physician about your fears on weight gain, or struggles with balanced food intake, and you may require more regular visits with your physician. I would recommend meeting with a dietitian who has experience with eating disorders to help with guidance and empower you to make solid food choices to aid in gaining or losing weight. Having structure with meal planning will help you if you are struggling with weight gain and weight loss. This will be a great way to create a foundation for if and when you do seek to get pregnant. I also encourage women who struggle with eating too much and too little to adopt a few techniques that stem from the practice of mindful eating on listening to hunger cues (feeling full or hungry), eating slowly without distractions, and appreciating your food." - Elizabeth Stanway-Mayers, Clinical Dietitian, Stanford University Medical Center

BONUS: Dental hygiene

You probably weren't expecting a book like this one to remind you get regular dental check-ups. Well, surprise! Your teeth and gums are practically the only area that your fertility doctor won't directly be asking about in the consultation, as that's a dentist's domain. Gum disease could mean deeper problems than just the superficial: it's been suggested that certain dental problems could equal inflammation, which could equal fertility issues. The CDC estimates that nearly half of American adults have mild, moderate or severe periodontitis, a gum condition that damages the soft tissue and destroys the bone that supports your teeth.[440] It's caused by poor oral hygiene. Researchers recommend that women of child bearing age should have regular preventive dental check-ups in order to maintain good oral and periodontal health.[441]

In summary...

- Three to four months before starting your ovarian stimulation cycle is a good amount of time to get Fertility Fit™.

- In general, the sooner you start making fertility-friendly lifestyle changes the better. Even if you only have a short period of time, every little bit counts.

- If you're medically considered overweight or underweight, or if you're a smoker, consider addressing these key lifestyle factors in good time before your egg freezing cycle.

- Focus on sustained changes over time rather than sudden, drastic ones, as these could even be counter-productive for your fertility

- Get a dental check-up.

Chapter 7: How Lifestyle Changes Can Affect Your Eggs

"Everything must be made as simple as possible. But not simpler."

— *Albert Einstein*

What exactly are the things you'll be attempting to improve with lifestyle changes? Without underplaying the deep complexity of how your ovaries produce eggs, there are three scientifically identified factors that influence the ability of your ovaries to produce quality eggs as you age. These are: oxidative stress, hormonal balance and energy production.

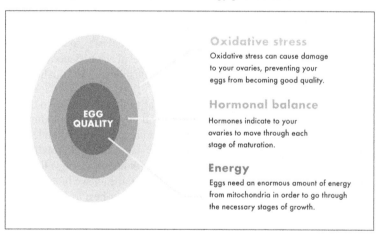

EGG QUALITY

Oxidative stress
Oxidative stress can cause damage to your ovaries, preventing your eggs from becoming good quality.

Hormonal balance
Hormones indicate to your ovaries to move through each stage of maturation.

Energy
Eggs need an enormous amount of energy from mitochondria in order to go through the necessary stages of growth.

Egg quality influencer 1: oxidative stress

Oxidative stress in your cells is caused by the overabundance of molecules called free radicals, which cause damage to the cells in your ovaries.[442] Free radicals are the natural byproducts, or waste products, from various chemical reactions such as metabolism. So the formation of some free radicals is a normal and inevitable process in the body. In fact, some super healthy activities like running can actually cause free radicals to form. However, when the number of free radicals in cells builds up unchecked, they start to be a problem. While also being associated with human diseases (such as cancer or Alzheimer's), free radicals are also linked to aging. Antioxidant levels are thought to play a crucial role in regulating many processes related to ageing, and in particular, reproduction.[443] Excessive oxidative stress on your ovaries is considered to be a contributing factor to various reproductive issues.[444] For example, it's tied to PCOS,[445] endometriosis,[446] preeclampsia,[447][448] recurrent miscarriage,[449] and it can even modulate age-related fertility decline by condensing your fertile years, causing early onset menopause.[450][451][452][453]

Scientists believe it poses a triple threat to your fertility by:

1. Dysregulating hormones [454]

2. Causing damage to energy-producing centers in cells (mitochondria) [455][456][457][458]

3. Causing DNA and cell damage [459]

These three forms of damage due to a build-up of oxidative stress can translate to two main negative outcomes for your egg freezing procedure. First, you might have fewer eggs retrieved. This is thought to happen because an abundance of free radicals essentially "kill off" some of the growing follicles before they make it to the retrieval stage. Second, of those eggs that are retrieved, fewer are likely to be considered good quality.[460][461][462][463][464][465]

So how can lifestyle changes help neutralize this? One way to defend against the damage caused by these free radical "fighters" is with the help of antioxidants. Having ample antioxidants can help create a suitable environment for your eggs during their fragile stages of rapid growth.

Substances that form free radicals can be found in the foods that we eat, the medicines and other substances we ingest, the air we breathe and the water we drink,[466] so we'll cover both how to do your best to avoid them in the world around you, and how to boost your antioxidant levels through diet and supplementation to keep them in check.

Egg quality influencer 2: imbalanced hormones

Reproduction as a whole is a finely tuned process run by a sophisticated balance of interacting hormones. These hormones work like a symphony orchestra, each playing a subtle role in concert with the others - so if one hormone plays out of tune, it can disrupt the entire performance. In other words, if the signals hormones send are disrupted, left unsent, or are unable to be received at any point while your eggs are growing, your ovaries won't receive the message to carry on with the key phases of chromosomal processing. Meaning: they won't become quality eggs.[467] [468] [469]

And, achieving the right balance of hormones needed to send the right signals is harder than you think, especially as you get older. As you age, your ovaries become less responsive to hormone messages from the brain, leaving more opportunities for disruption.[470]

Egg quality influencer 3: energy production

Your growing eggs need an incredible amount of energy to get safely through all the stages of chromosomal processing. They get this energy from mitochondria, which are the tiny "power plants" in your cells.[471] While mitochondria are contained in almost every cell in your body,[472] in your eggs there are more than ten times the number found in any other cell (there are about 100,000 mitochondria in one fully-grown human egg).[473] That's a testament to how energy intensive it is to mature your eggs. Even the follicle surrounding your egg has its own mitochondria, which are known to give your egg an extra power boost when needed.[474] In fact, it's now thought that the ability of mitochondria to effectively create a substance called ATP (cell energy) when it is needed is the single most important factor in determining the viability of eggs and embryos.[475]

As you age, your mitochondria decline both in quantity and in power supply, similar to the fading capabilities of an AA battery.[476] By the time you hit 40, almost one-third of the mitochondria in your eggs will no longer be efficient energy producers.[477] And when this happens, there isn't enough energy to fuel egg maturation and chromosomal processing, which often results in low quality eggs.[478] [479] [480] [481] [482] [483] [484] [485] What is amazing is that scientists now believe that, whilst your mitochondria are like batteries, they're more like the rechargeable kind. Certain supplements may be able to give them a power boost and there are some key lifestyle choices you can make to protect them from damage - all of which we'll be covering in the upcoming chapters.

Chapter 8: Eating for Egg Health

"You are what you eat, so don't be fast, cheap, easy, or fake."

-Anonymous

According to researchers, optimizing your diet before treatment could not only improve egg quality and your reproductive health, but it could also increase your mental health and reduce costs.[486] Eating for egg health is not a fad aimed at making you look a certain way, but rather, it's a way of reframing your relationship with food so you can get your developing eggs into the best possible shape before the big retrieval day. This comes from evidence indicating that the foods you eat can have a profound effect on the maturation, development and quality of your eggs.[487 488 489 490] In fact, what you eat is so instrumental that some scientists believe that nearly half of *all* cases of infertility are due to improper nutrition.[491] That's pretty incredible.

So, you'd be correct if you already deduced that eating healthily overall would be good for your eggs. However, there are some dietary additions and exclusions that are known to be *particularly* beneficial to your eggs and ovaries - some of them even counterintuitive. So, try not to be tempted to skip this section even if you already know your kale from your quinoa.

What the science says about food and your fertility

There is resounding evidence that food affects a variety of bodily processes that are essential for optimal fertility. The right foods help you:

- **Maintain hormonal balance** - Reproductive hormones are synthesized in the body by proteins and fats from food.[492 493 494 495]

- **Limit oxidative stress** - A poor diet with lots of fried and processed foods can cause oxidative stress around your eggs and ovaries, while some foods have antioxidants that can help protect against it.[496]

- **Supply essential nutrients** - Key proteins oversee DNA processing during egg maturation,[497] many of which can only come from dietary sources.[498 499 500]

- **Regulate sleep patterns** - Dietary patterns may help regulate sleep and improve sleep quality, which can affect your hormones and ovulation.[501]

- **Boost cell energy** - Compounds in certain foods fuel your mitochondria.[502]

- **Help you maintain optimal weight** - A balanced, nutrient-rich diet with healthy fats can help maintain fertility-friendly bodyweight (BMI of 20-25).[503 504 505 506]

- **Stabilize blood sugar levels** - Elevated blood sugar levels caused by foods with a high glycemic load (GL) can cause ovulatory dysfunction.[507 508 509]

- **Regulate stress** - Diets low in sugar and junk food are linked to better moods. And the relationship goes the other way, too. The stress hormone cortisol triggers blood sugar and insulin levels to rise in order to give you the energy to "fight or flight" from a stressful situation. When you are chronically stressed, this can lead to insulin resistance,[510 511] which disrupts the balance of hormones needed to properly mature your eggs.[512 513 514]

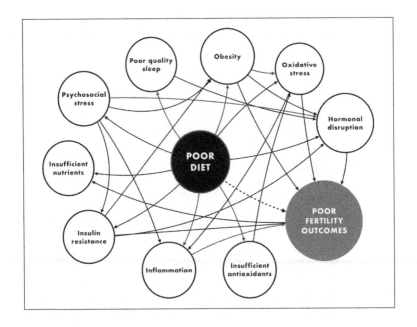

Can't I just take a supplement?

If there was one pill that would deliver all the sustenance needed for quality eggs (whilst keeping us at a fertility-friendly weight, with a healthy gut etc. etc…) we'd be all over it. Alas, there is not.

For the most part, the nutrients derived from food are simply superior to their synthetic cousins. When you eat real food, you're not consuming single nutrients, but rather a whole range of vitamins, minerals, enzymes, carotenoids, flavonoids and antioxidants that enable optimal use by the body.[515] [516] [517] For example, the antioxidant activity in a small apple is equivalent to what you would get from a huge slew of vitamin C (like, 1500 mg), despite the fact that the apple contains a smaller amount (5.7 mg) of the vitamin. That's because nearly all of the antioxidant power from apples is derived from a variety of other surrounding compounds or phytochemicals that work to enhance vitamin C's effect.[518] Nutrition is more complex than a set of baseline, static numbers, it also covers nuanced interactions between compounds. All the various compounds can join forces, neutralize each other and jostle for dominance.

Although this means you should take a "food first" approach when it comes to getting enough of certain nutrients, it's not always possible through food alone. For instance, food alone is not sufficient if you have a restricted diet (e.g. meat-focused, vegan, vegetarian, food allergies, or religious), if you have a malabsorptive condition or if you are already radically deficient in something - even if you are taking oral contraceptives, which can affect the absorption of certain vitamins and minerals. If this sounds like you, taking a supplement to top up the vitamins or antioxidants you'd normally get from food can be a solution. We'll cover more on this in the "Supplementing your Diet" chapter.

Twelve dietary tips to get Fertility Fit™

1. Buy foods closest to their natural form

Hint: flavored candy in the shape of fruit does not count. The most basic thing you can do each week to aid your fertility is to fill your grocery cart with minimally modified foods without any explicitly added or fortified ingredients (e.g. added salt, sugar, or vitamins).[519] So put anything from a box, jar, wrapper, can, bag or fast food window back on the shelf and head instead to the produce and refrigerated sections of the grocery store.

No matter how healthy most processed and fast foods profess to be - the marketing is almost terrifyingly good - don't be fooled. As we all probably already know (but like to let ourselves conveniently forget when faced with them), they are often filled with additives, sugar and saturated fat and are associated with poorer fertility outcomes.[520] One study found that regularly eating fast food (burgers, fried chicken, pizza, fries, etc.) was linked to a twofold increase in the risk of infertility.[521] Sticking to the fresh food sections, often located on the periphery of the grocery store, will help you adopt a "low processed" approach to consumption. Dutch researchers found that women who took this approach - eating fewer snack foods, meat and mayonnaise, and more legumes, vegetables, whole grains, and fish - were 40% more likely to get pregnant when trying than those that didn't.[522]

Not only will eating fried foods, processed products and baked goods make it difficult to maintain a fertility-friendly bodyweight,[523 524 525 526 527] but the cans and plastics surrounding packaged foods are likely to be laden with harmful chemicals like Bisphenol-A (BPA), which can disrupt your hormones and the maturation of your eggs (we'll cover more on this and other environmental nasties later).[528 529 530]

ELANZA PERSPECTIVE: "We are both partial (read: totally addicted) to potato chips: salty, laden with oil, fried...so bad, but so good. Rather than just cut all the joy from our lives, when we're at our desks and really craving these snacks we'll try to opt for a healthier replacement that still gives us our fix. Try freshly made popcorn, or lightly salted pumpkin seeds. Surprisingly hits the spot." - Brittany and Catherine

2. Buy the best whole foods you can afford

There isn't direct evidence that links any one type of farming practice to better fertility outcomes. However, meat and vegetables that are organic, free range, biodynamic, hormone free, etc. *are* less likely to be exposed to pesticides, which are known to disrupt hormones and cause damage to your cells.[531] There is also a higher likelihood that animals have been fed a more nutritious diet, and in turn, you can benefit from those nutrients too.[532]

When it comes to buying fruits and vegetables, there are a few where it really pays to buy organic. The Environmental Working Group has identified the most pesticide-laden twelve fruit and veg, also known as "The Dirty Dozen."[533] If financial or other restrictions mean you're not regularly able to buy these twelve fruits and veg organic, be extra careful to wash them very thoroughly before cooking or consuming them, to try to remove most of the surface pesticides. Or, instead, select fruit and veg from the "Clean 15" list of the produce with the lowest levels of pesticide exposure. Basically, don't avoid eating fruit or vegetables, just finesse your choices as best as possible. Check out the chart below to see what they are:

EWG 2019 Dirty Dozen	EWG 2019 Clean Fifteen
1. Strawberries	1. Avocados
2. Spinach	2. Sweet corn
3. Kale	3. Pineapples
4. Nectarines	4. Sweet peas
5. Apples	5. Onions
6. Grapes	6. Papayas
7. Peaches	7. Eggplants
8. Cherries	8. Asparagus
9. Pears	9. Kiwis
10. Tomatoes	10. Cabbages
11. Celery	11. Cauliflower
12. Potatoes	12. Cantaloupes
+ Hot peppers	13. Broccoli
	14. Mushrooms
	15. Honeydew melons

We'll discuss more on how to avoid pesticides further in the "Avoiding Hazards for Egg Health" chapter.

EXPERT INSIGHT: "If cost is a factor in accessing organic produce, consider purchasing them frozen. They are typically frozen shortly after harvest, when nutrients and taste are at their peak. The freezing process helps protect antioxidant and nutrient levels as well, so you don't necessarily need to think of the frozen section as inferior from a health perspective. You can save money buying frozen fruits and vegetables, especially when they're out of season (like frozen berries in the dead of winter). When buying fresh fruits and vegetables, research what is in season in your area; those choices tend to be more nutrient-dense, better tasting, and less expensive than out of season produce that's been shipped from across the world." - Kaitlyn Noble, Pre and Post-natal Health Coach, Los Angeles

2. Mix up your meals

Adequate nutrient levels provide the foundation for optimal fertility. Adding a variety of ingredients to each and every meal sets you up to get the full span of the nutrients you need to support your egg health, and helps your body to make the most of them. Eating the same foods all the time can surprisingly easily lead to deficiencies in some vitamins and minerals, while overloading you with others. It can even overexpose you to other environmental toxins such as pesticides and BPA plastics, things that are found in the cultivation or production of those foods. So, no matter how healthily you think you're eating, you really can get too much of a good thing.

A cautionary tale of too much kale

Cast your mind back to the height of kale stardom when some people, even the actor Jake Gyllenhaal, took up all-kale diets.[534] People were making everything out of kale in hopes that this nutrition powerhouse would solve all of life's problems.[535] When San Francisco-based molecular biologist Ernie Hubbard started hearing about a wave of otherwise super healthy people complaining about experiencing chronic fatigue, foggy thinking, skin and hair issues, arrhythmias and neurological disorders, he set out to find the culprit. It turns out that they all had high levels of a substance called thallium in their blood. Hubbard suspects that this came from excessive consumption of kale, but also other veggies like cabbage and cauliflower. That's because these vegetables are particularly adept at soaking up thallium from soil, which could potentially lead to a form of metal poisoning. The moral of the story is: vary your veggies.

Another benefit of eating a variety of "real" foods in one meal is that your body can make the most out of the available nutrients because the nutrients in most foods are complemented by the nutrients in others. The way in which our bodies absorb and process nutrients is a big puzzle with many pieces that slot together.

For example, these "power couples" from different food sources work closely together and interact, meaning a deficiency of one could halt the proper functioning of the other:

- Vitamin B12 and folate
- Vitamin D and calcium
- Zinc and copper

Food variation challenge:
An easy way to pack lots of complementary nutrients into one meal is to eat salads, soups and stir-frys. Challenge yourself by trying to include all colors of the rainbow in just one dish. We find that this way of thinking helps us feel fuller and more satisfied, and leaves us with fewer cravings for the other stuff.

3. Maximize vitamins and minerals

Did you know that vitamins and minerals of all sorts can be found in abundance inside your ovaries?[536] [537] [538] While this is a growing area of research, it's safe to say that most vitamins, minerals, and antioxidants play some role in the process of preparing your body and your eggs for reproduction, whether it's directly or indirectly. Let's take a closer look at some of the key vitamins and minerals from food that researchers have identified as having a direct impact on fertility:

Folate (AKA Folic Acid or Vitamin B9)

Folate has long been considered an integral vitamin for pregnancy as it can help reduce the likelihood of certain birth defects.[539] But new research reveals that it also plays a crucial role in ovulation and maturation of your eggs. Folate plays a few important roles in fertility: it is responsible for making new copies of DNA and for making the building blocks of proteins, both of which are important in early egg development.[540] [541] Additionally, folate is known to prevent an amino acid called homocysteine from building up in your body. When high concentrations of this acid are detected in a woman's body, she is likely to have fewer, lower quality eggs retrieved from IVF cycles compared to women that don't have elevated levels.[542] [543] [544]

Further evidence for the importance of folate comes from a study that found that women who take folic acid supplements before going through IVF had higher quality eggs and a higher proportion of mature eggs than women that did not take the additional folate.[545] Yet another study found that women with twice the amount of folate measured in the follicular fluid surrounding their eggs were three times more likely to become pregnant.[546]

Here's the rub: your body cannot create its own folate, nor can it be stored in your body. This is why you should aim to eat folate-rich foods every day. That said, experts believe it is "almost impossible" to get the recommended 600 micrograms (.6mg) of folic acid per day just from food, which is why taking a folic acid supplement is also commonly advised.[547] We'll discuss this further in the "Supplementing your Diet" chapter.

Food sources for folate: *Spinach, broccoli, avocado, brussels sprouts, artichoke, asparagus, lentils and other beans.*[548]

Vitamin B12

To emphasize the importance of this vitamin, consider that pregnant women with B12 deficiencies are at a high risk of spontaneous abortion. People with vitamin B12 deficiencies often have high concentrations of harmful homocysteine in their bloodstreams as well. Vitamin B12 has been shown to work together with vitamins B6 and folic acid (see above) to control elevated blood levels of homocysteine,[549] which can influence your egg freezing outcome. A study also associated high levels of B12 in the follicular fluid surrounding the egg with better embryo quality from women undergoing IVF.[550] B12 deficiency is fairly common, and, although in many cases the cause of the deficiency is actually unknown, reasons can include malabsorption from food. That's why oral dietary supplements or injections may be necessary[551] [552]

Food sources for vitamin B12: *Clams, oysters, mussels, liver, caviar (fish eggs), fish, crab, lobster, beef, lamb, dairy, cheese, eggs.*[553]

EXPERT INSIGHT: "This is particularly important for vegans and vegetarians, since B12 is primarily found in animal sources. Fortified nutritional yeast is an excellent source of B12 if you don't consume animal products." - Kaitlyn Noble, Pre and Post-natal Health Coach, Los Angeles

Zinc

Zinc is increasingly being identified as an important player in the process of maturing quality eggs, as well as the other half of the equation, sperm. A 2018 study conducted on mice indicates that having a zinc deficiency could negatively affect the early stages of egg development by reducing the ability of the egg cells to divide and be fertilized. The researchers said their findings showed that zinc plays a role in egg growth at an earlier stage than previously investigated - which is to say, actually *during development* and before division. That's the stage most of your eggs are at right now. They also pointed out that the eggs collected in ovarian stimulation cycles are taken from mature (antral) follicles, at which point the zinc effects have already occurred."[554] In other words, getting plenty of zinc in the few months prior to your retrieval, while your eggs are still developing, could be super important.

Zinc has also been found to be a crucial presence later on in the various stages of egg maturation. One study even found that eggs need a 50% extra boost in zinc in order to reach full maturity. The "flood" of zinc to the egg is believed to push the egg into the final stages of egg maturation.[555] [556] [557] [558] [559] The World Health Organization estimates that 17% of the global population is vulnerable to zinc deficiency. [560] Although this includes women all around the world, including those with limited diets, it's still worth being extra diligent about making sure you get enough zinc by eating plenty of the right foods.

Food sources for zinc: *Oysters, beef, turkey, darker meats, other shellfish, beans, pumpkin seeds, nuts, whole grains, dairy products.*[561] *Zinc is best eaten with foods that contain sulfur: garlic, onion, whole eggs.*

Vitamin B6

Women with low levels of vitamin B6 may be less likely to become pregnant and more likely to miscarry (which can be a sign of low egg quality). When the researchers in one study provided B6 supplements, conception increased by 40% and early miscarriage decreased by 30%.[562] It's not known whether this is due to changes to the quality of the egg, uterus or both, but either way, it's not harmful to eat lots of vitamin B6-rich foods and may help mature the best possible eggs, so for us it's a no-brainer.

Food sources for vitamin B6: *Tuna, bananas, turkey, liver, salmon, cod, spinach, bell peppers, and turnip greens, collard greens, garlic, cauliflower, mustard greens, celery, cabbage, asparagus, broccoli, kale, brussels sprouts, swiss chard.*[563]

Vitamin D (AKA Calciferol)

In the past decade, vitamin D has become a hot area of research; low levels of vitamin D have now been implicated in a wide variety of diseases, including diabetes, cancer, obesity, multiple sclerosis, arthritis, as well as all kinds of fertility related issues.[564] Vitamin D deficiency can even have an impact on your mental health and happiness (which you'll want to be extra aware of during the emotional peaks and valleys that can occur during the hormonal stimulation phase).[565]

While studies on the direct association between vitamin D levels and pregnancy are mixed,[566] [567] [568] [569] [570] we do know that vitamin D plays a role in producing reproductive hormones, which provides a clue as to the seriousness of this deficiency. What you may not know is that, contrary to its name, vitamin D isn't really a vitamin at all. It's actually a fat soluble hormone itself.[571] Because of the knock-on effect hormones have on each other, researchers believe that having too little vitamin D can interrupt or alter your body's production of estrogen, progesterone, anti-Müllerian hormone (AMH) and follicle stimulation hormone (FSH), all of which are involved in the growth of your ovarian follicles.[572] [573] Further research has shown that there are specific receptors for vitamin D in cells in the ovaries and the womb, which has led scientists to believe it plays some role in reproduction but further studies are needed.[574]

Despite the currently inconclusive evidence on vitamin D and fertility, it's worth mentioning because over a third of the US population is considered vitamin D deficient.[575] [576] Even though it is possible to obtain small amounts of vitamin D from food, the vast majority of vitamin D in the body is generated by exposure to ultraviolet B (UVB) exposure from sunlight.[577] Given the widespread (and valid) public health messaging around using sunscreen, plus the rise of indoor desk jobs and pursuits (video games, box sets, Instagram addiction), it's not surprising that many people aren't getting enough rays. We're not suggesting switching off Netflix entirely - you actually only need around 10-30 minutes of sunlight a few times a week to maintain healthy blood levels if you're Caucasian. If you have darker skin, (African-American, or of south Asian origin) then you'll need to spend longer in the sun for the same effect - and you should be particularly mindful of deficiency.

In the winter, the sunlight in a lot of states (and many northern hemisphere countries) doesn't contain enough UVB radiation for your skin to be able to make vitamin D from it. So, during these months make particular effort to eat vitamin D-rich foods (including fortified foods) to get your dose. Incidentally, sitting by a sunny window won't cut it - the UVB won't get through glass. Sunbeds can work, but they're not recommended as a way of making vitamin B because of the link with skin cancer.

Adequate vitamin D levels are considered within the 25–40 ng/mL range. If you want to check your levels, you can request a blood test from your doctor or you can order an at-home test kit.

Food sources for vitamin D: *Spinach, broccoli, avocado, brussels sprouts, artichoke, asparagus, lentils and other beans.*[578]

4. Add in antioxidants

A growing amount of research indicates that upping your intake of antioxidants can help combat oxidative stress by neutralizing harmful free radicals.[579][580] Getting antioxidants through food, compared to supplements, offers them up in ideal proportions and combinations that dispose, scavenge, or suppress the formation of free radicals that cause harmful oxidative stress. Getting antioxidants through food also ensures appropriate absorption because of the other minerals that help drive those essential vitamins into the cells (i.e. magnesium helps your body absorb vitamin D. And methylated folate, as well as other B vitamins, are ingested in their most active form through food.)

DOCTOR INSIGHT: "There have been some studies which suggest that an increase in antioxidants may also be beneficial to egg quality." – Dr. Peter Klatsky, Spring Fertility, San Francisco

This should be of particular note if you have PCOS, as women with the condition tend to have lower antioxidant measurements compared to other women.[581][582] However, scientists still don't have a complete understanding of how they act in our bodies.

Antioxidants are in all kinds of foods we eat because every plant[583] and animal has its own unique antioxidant defenses needed to fight off free radicals - many of which we can only get by eating them. Some of the key antioxidants that are tied to egg health are: melatonin,[584] selenium,[585] vitamin E,[586] and vitamin C,[587] lipoic acid[588] and beta-carotene.[589] Structuring your meals to be full of antioxidants might be particularly something to focus on if you are older than thirty because as you age, your body has fewer natural antioxidant defenses, which leaves more free radicals the opportunity to damage the DNA of your delicate eggs.[590][591]

Food sources for antioxidants: *Goji berries, blueberries, dark chocolate, pecans, artichoke, blackberries, sweet potatoes, carrots, squash, broccoli, asparagus, mushrooms, green leafy vegetables, red peppers, cabbage, potatoes, tomatoes, and citrus fruit. Meat and eggs contain some antioxidants, which are mainly from the nutrient-rich plants the animals fed on. That said, grass fed meat and dairy products as well as eggs from pastured hens rank higher in terms of their antioxidant count.*

Herbs and spices are also a great source of antioxidants: *Cilantro, cloves, cinnamon, oregano, turmeric, cumin, parsley, basil, ginger, thyme.*

Best eaten with healthy fats: *Grass-fed butter, olive oil, coconut oil, nuts, avocado to help the nutrients absorb better because they are fat-soluble vitamins.*

5. Get less of your protein from meat

We all know it's important to get enough protein in our diets, but does it matter what kind? A growing body of research suggests that not all proteins are created equal, and not in the way you might assume. Generally vegetarians come in for a bit of a grilling (excuse the pun) when the topic of protein is raised, but, interestingly, carnivores might do well to pay attention, too. A diet that is high in red meat may impact fertility, researchers say.[592] That might be, they say, due to the presence in meat of compounds known as - rather appropriately in this context - AGE (advanced glycation end-products).[593] [594] The accumulation of these compounds in women's bodies has been highly correlated with poor follicular development (as well as poor embryo development and miscarriage).[595] [596] If you eat a lot of red meat, you could try replacing some dishes with different protein sources, such as prawns, fish or crab. It's thought that a diet high in seafood (with all those omega fatty acids) may help improve fertility.[597] In fact, one study of women undergoing ART cycles found that the ones who ate more fish were up to 50% more likely to have a baby, compared to those who ate other protein sources such as red meat.[598]

A bit of background: protein rich foods such as meat, fish, dairy, beans and legumes are broken down into 20 different types of amino acids, some of which are synthesized into hormones and enzymes that are vital to your reproductive health.[599] While your body can synthesize eleven amino acids by itself, the other nine *must* come from dietary sources. Proteins that contain these nine amino acids are called "complete proteins." A common misconception is that vegetarians and vegans cannot get complete proteins through a non-animal diet and that, therefore, these diets cannot be healthy. But, don't worry, that's not based on fact. Optimizing your diet for reproduction needn't mean sacrificing your religious beliefs, values or personal preferences. Contrary to what we often hear, you *can* also get complete proteins from non-animal sources, for example, quinoa and buckwheat, which are both complete proteins. You can also mix different types of plant protein in one meal to construct your own complete protein, for instance, pairing rice and beans/legumes, or pita and hummus together, as is common practice in countries and cultures where vegetarians are in the majority, such as India. You don't need every single amino acid in one mouthful - if you get the full set across the day, your body will do the rest.

Even if you do eat meat, a study suggests it could be beneficial to your fertility to replace some animal protein from your diet with vegetable protein (beans, legumes, nuts and seeds) - researchers say by doing this you could reduce the risk of ovulatory infertility by more than 50%, especially if you are over 32 years old.[600]

As American women in their 30s are generally consuming at the very top end of recommended meat consumption levels, it's worth considering making some healthier protein choices across some of your meals.[601] Overall, advice for a relatively sedentary woman is to consume 0.36 grams of protein a day per pound of body weight (calculation: 0.36 x your body weight in lbs), which makes the guideline amount to aim for around 46 grams per day. However, bear in mind that this number fluctuates based on your age and activity level. The United States Department of Agriculture (USDA) has a handy daily intake calculator that combines all these factors: https://fnic.nal.usda.gov/fnic/dri-calculator/index.php. For reference (as it's near impossible to picture actual foods from these measures!) a standard three ounce serving of cooked salmon will give you 19 grams of protein, around half your daily intake.[602] Beans are also a high source of protein, containing around 12 grams of protein in a one cup serving.[603]

Added bonus: plant protein tends to be cheaper, more nutrient dense, lower in calories and saturated fat, and higher in fiber!

Even plant protein pumps up the iron

Women sometimes worry that cutting out red meat might lead to an iron deficiency, but iron is also available from non-meat sources such as broccoli, lentils, beans and cashews, or in supplements. It's important to make sure you eat enough of these iron-rich foods, both for your reproductive health and possibly for egg health. Not only has iron from plants ("non-heme" iron) been linked to a reduction in ovulatory infertility[604] but one recent study indicates the potential role of iron in the cultivation of quality eggs, specifically in the role it plays in the process of providing oxygen to the ovaries. Good flow of fresh, oxygenated blood to the ovaries is important for egg development.[605]

Food sources for iron: *Lentils, spinach, sesame seeds, kidney beans, pumpkin seeds (raw), venison, garbanzo beans, navy beans, seaweed, beef, pork.*[606]

EXPERT INSIGHT: "Well-designed vegetarian diets are appropriate for all stages of life, including pregnancy and lactation, according to the Academy of Nutrition and Dietetics. It is crucial to eat enough of a variety of good protein-containing sources from diverse plant-based foods." - Elizabeth Stanway-Mayers, Clinical Dietitian, Stanford University Medical Center

How about protein from soy?

Soy's effect on fertility has stirred up a bit of debate over the years. Soy contains compounds called "isoflavones" which are also called "phytoestrogens" as they behave like estrogens in your body. That's why soy isoflavones have been tested for use as hormone replacement therapy in menopause. And, as such, it's thought they have the potential to impact fertility.[607] [608]

While the research is still limited and difficult to measure, some researchers believe this estrogenic activity might have a negative impact on your ovarian function.[609] However, far from some of the scare stories we read in the media, most of the evidence points to soy actually being *good* for fertility. Evidence for the positive benefits of soy come from multiple studies which found that women who either ate ample soy in their diet or took soy supplements prior to ART treatment had higher fertilization rates, clinical pregnancies, and live births versus those that didn't.[610] [611] [612] There could be confounding factors, for instance, those eating more soy may also have generally healthier diets, eating lots of vegetables, too. However, a study on mice in a more controlled environment indicated benefits too. The results associate dietary intake of soy with improved egg quality.[613]

The takeaway here is that there isn't conclusive evidence whether soy is good or bad for you, or even if it has any tangible effect at all. All the headlines generate a lot of noise, but not a great deal is actually being said. What *is* the case, though, is that soy is one of the most commonly genetically modified crops, and it's likely to have been inundated with toxic pesticides (a big alarm bell for fertility, as we'll discover).

EXPERT INSIGHT: "Choose whole sources of soy like organic edamame, tempeh, or tofu and limit processed sources like 'fake' meats, protein powders, and health bars." - Kaitlyn Noble, Pre and Post-natal Health Coach, Los Angeles

6. Adopt "Mediterranean fats" into your diet

Fat consumption is one of the most hotly debated dietary issues of our lifetimes.[614] The official advice on fat over the last 100 years has dramatically switched gears, as the science has evolved.[615] [616] One absolutely critical thing to understand (especially if you've been raised to be fat-phobic), is that some fat in your diet is *essential* to good reproductive health.[617] That's because fats regulate the production of reproductive hormones.

But before you dive into that side of streaky bacon, you should know that not all fats are equally good for your fertility. Studies have identified that *polyunsaturated* fats, in specific amounts, are beneficial and should replace saturated fats in your diet, which are not beneficial.[618]

That's not to say you shouldn't have any saturated fat or cholesterol - they play a role, too. Cholesterol is a precursor to all hormones produced in the body, including progesterone.[619] The key is to make sure you select the right source foods to limit your saturated fat and aim for the *good* types of cholesterol, rather than bad: for example, fish, nuts, seeds and some coconut oil and grass-fed meats. Avoid other sources of saturated fat and cholesterol, such as hydrogenated oils and vegetable oils, especially when fried or cooked at high temperatures.

One category of fat you should avoid entirely is "trans fats." These are most often found in commercial baked and fried foods, such as doughnuts and cookies. They are man-made fats created to increase a product's shelf life and allow oil to be reused after it has been heated. If you live in the US, Denmark, Switzerland or Austria that should be pretty simple, as the authorities have now banned trans fats. But if you live in the UK, North Africa, the Middle East, or South Asia, make sure you read the labels (or better yet, avoid packaged foods entirely), as at the time of writing trans fat are still legally allowed in many snack foods.

A great shorthand way to aim for the "good" fats is to eat a Mediterranean-inspired diet. The Mediterranean diet - rich in vegetables, fish, nuts and seeds, and olive oil - is the most widely researched dietary pattern for reproductive benefits in the world.[620] [621] [622] Studies have found all sorts of benefits of eating this way, for example:

- Couples undergoing IVF were more likely to get pregnant when they incorporated a Mediterranean diet six months before treatment.[623]

- Women who followed a Mediterranean-style diet while trying to conceive had a 66% lower risk of ovulation problems and a 27% lower risk of infertility due to other causes, compared to those who didn't follow the diet. This is according to the largest study on fertility ever done! [624]

- Women with Mediterranean diets have been shown to have improved egg quality, embryo growth, and pregnancy rates, and time to pregnancy.[625] [626] [627] [628] [629]

- Research even indicates that men who follow the Mediterranean diet are able to improve their semen quality.[630]

DOCTOR INSIGHT: "Monounsaturated and polyunsaturated fats are great regulators in the production of reproductive hormones whereas saturated fats cause increases in homocysteine levels which then leads to increased inflammation in the body. Healthy fats have also been found to regulate cortisol levels and satiate cravings which may provide a hypothesis as to why women who ate Mediterranean diets rich in monounsaturated and polyunsaturated fats experienced improved rates of fertility." - Dr. Hemalee Patel, Lifestyle Medicine Expert, San Francisco

---

Cooking with oil
EXPERT PERSPECTIVE: "While olive oil is a fantastic way to get healthy fats when incorporated into salads and seasonings, it's not always the best choice if used in a hot pan. When olive oil gets really hot it often smokes, oxidizes and becomes toxic. When I roast vegetables, I prefer to use ghee because it can hold up to the heat and still provides a slew of nutrients. As a rule of thumb, olive oil and most other plant-based oils are excellent served cold or for light sauteing, while ghee or avocado oil are better for higher heat cooking." - Kaitlyn Noble, Pre and Post-natal Health Coach, Los Angeles

---

Cut down on saturated fats

In contrast to the Mediterranean diet, foods full of saturated fats such as coconut oil, mayonnaise, butter, and red meat have shown to have a negatively affect egg development, embryo quality and pregnancy rates.[631] [632] [633] That doesn't mean you can never eat them, but the advice is to consume them less frequently.

What's the deal with dairy?

A common source of saturated fat is from dairy foods like butter and cheese. You might hear some people extolling the virtues of a dairy-free diet, while others call it a key "fertility food." So what's the reality? Well, dairy is a tricky subject when it comes to fertility, because research on the subject is limited and inconsistent.[634] [635] [636] [637] [638]

Basically, of the limited studies, many show conflicting results.[639] Based on some of the evidence, you might come across a fertility doctor who recommends adding "a bowl of full fat ice cream" a day to boost reproductive function (we're all ears...). This advice comes from a study that followed the diets of more than 18,000 women over an eight year time frame. The study found that the women who ate more high fat dairy products had a lower risk of ovulatory infertility, whereas women who consumed more low-fat dairy (including skim, 1%, and 2% milk, yogurt, or cottage cheese) were at a higher risk.[640] Then again, other studies have not found this to be true.[641] [642] The thing is, there could be other differentiating lifestyle choices between women who ate full fat dairy products and those who opted for skim versions. It's hard to look at the impact of dairy as having an effect.

Without sufficient evidence leaning heavily in one direction or the other, the best thing you can do is read your own body and pay attention to how consuming dairy makes you feel. One thing you should watch out for is heavily processed dairy products, especially those with sneaky amounts of added sugar (more on that in a minute). There's always some naturally occurring sugar (lactose) in dairy, which is OK. OK, that is, unless you are allergic or intolerant - then, take advice from a doctor or other specialist about what is recommended for you. If you choose to eat dairy and have no problems digesting it, just try to still think in terms of "whole" and "natural" versions - watch out for high amounts of corn syrup and cane sugar on the ingredients list, especially in flavored yogurts and ice creams.

DOCTOR PERSPECTIVE: "When patients ask me if they should cut down dairy I go through the evidence and let them know there is increasing evidence to suggest that dairy can cause low levels of inflammation in the body that can affect fertility. I will often ask my patients after they eat dairy to notice if they tend to get dry skin, worsening eczema/dandruff, runny nose, worsening allergies, puffy eyes or swollen, achy or stiff joints the day after ingesting. If they answer yes to any of these it can suggest a mild allergic response which may be something they want to avoid when going through fertility treatments, as we know any low level of inflammation can affect reproductive health." - Dr. Hemalee Patel, Lifestyle Medicine Expert, San Francisco

EXPERT INSIGHT: "With regards to that 'extra bowl of ice cream' advice - ice cream is made from dairy and has some calcium. The correct serving size is half of a cup, but, let's be honest...most of us eat more. There are other healthier options to help reach your calcium and fat quota. For someone who is trying to lose weight, I would recommend other foods higher in calcium over ice cream such as milk, cheese, yogurt, canned fish, dark leafy greens, soybeans, and enriched cereal/grains. On the other hand, if someone is actively trying to gain weight, ice cream would be an appropriate food choice in terms of calories for weight gain." - Elizabeth Stanway-Mayers, Clinical Dietitian, Stanford University Medical Center

Balance out your omegas

A major plus of the Mediterranean diet is that it includes many foods that are abundant in omega-3 fatty acids - the ones we all tend to need more of - and is lower in omega-6s, the ones we all get enough of and might need to be mindful to limit.

Omega-6 overload
Human beings evolved on a diet with a ratio of 1:1 omega 3 to 6 and now our diets have a ratio of between 1:10 to 1:25![643] The spike in omega-6 happened as vegetable oils were added to all kinds of foods and cereal grains were fed to domestic livestock, altering the fat profile of meat.[644]

While we're generally wary of the term "superfood," omega-3s can genuinely be considered a fertility super building-block. The power of omega-3 in relation to fertility is thought to be tied to its ability to reduce inflammation, manage insulin levels in response to glucose,[645] support progesterone production, and increase blood flow to the reproductive organs.[646]

On the other hand, omega-6s are thought to be pro-inflammatory, causing oxidative stress on our bodies, including our reproductive system. One study conducted on mice even indicated that even *short-term* dietary treatment with a diet rich in omega-3 fatty acids is associated with improved egg quality, while short-term dietary treatment with omega-6 fatty acids results in very poor egg quality. The researchers determined that "omega-3 fatty acids may provide an effective and practical avenue for delaying ovarian aging and improving egg quality at advanced maternal age."[647] [648] This is exciting news for your fertility all around!

Omega-3 food sources: *The best, most absorbable form is found in fatty, cold-water fish such as salmon, trout, cod, herring, mackerel, and sardines, and in shellfish such as shrimp, oysters, clams, and scallops. Omega-3 can be found in plant sources such as flax seeds, hemp, chia seeds, and raw walnuts, but it is not absorbed as well.[649] A good rule of thumb is using olive oil for salads and other cold dishes, butter for baking and roasting and rapeseed oil (a healthy version of canola oil, low in saturated fat) for everything else. Note that in the US canola oil tends to be GMO and processed - you might have to do a bit of searching to find "cold pressed" or unprocessed canola oil.*

Reducing omega-6s: *Avoid more refined vegetable oils. If you eat red meat, make it organic and grass-fed and if you eat chicken, go for organic and free-range.*

Be mindful of mercury

While fish and shellfish can offer a variety of nutritional benefits, you might reconsider the types that you eat and in what amount. This is because fish and shellfish are exposed to low concentrations of mercury from water pollution, which accumulate in their bodies over time. This highly toxic form of mercury, called methylmercury, can cause serious health issues if it gets to certain levels in your body, and could have implications for your fertility. For example, one study conducted in Hong Kong (where seafood comes from highly polluted waters) found that men and women with "unexplained infertility" had higher concentrations of mercury in their bloodstreams than women without fertility issues. The amount of mercury in their bloodstreams also aligned with the amount of seafood in their diets.[650]

As a rule of thumb, you can presume that larger and longer-lived fish tend to contain higher levels of mercury.[651] Larger fish tend to eat many smaller fish, which contain small amounts of mercury[652] and longer-lived fish have accumulated mercury over time.

Foods with mercury to avoid: *Shark, swordfish, tilefish, and king mackerel. Albacore tuna also contains a moderate amount of mercury and should not be eaten more than once per week. Canned light tuna is relatively low in mercury.*

7. Stabilize your blood sugar levels

Your blood sugar level has an effect on just about every aspect of your reproductive system, so not surprisingly it also includes the health of your eggs. How does this translate to the outcome of your egg freezing procedure? Evidence points to reductions in both the quality and quantity of eggs retrieved. For example, a study on women undergoing IVF found that the women who had higher blood sugar levels over time had fewer eggs retrieved, fewer eggs fertilized, and fewer good-quality embryos.[653] And if we look at the effects of blood sugar on your long term reproductive health, research indicates that even slightly higher blood glucose levels can reduce the chance of a natural pregnancy by more than 50%.[654]

The science behind blood sugar
The primary issue is related to insulin, a hormone that plays a crucial role in helping your body convert sugars into energy. It removes excess glucose (sugar) from your blood and packs it into your liver, muscles, and fat cells to be used as energy later. The more sugar you ingest, the more insulin your body has to create in order to maintain your blood sugar level. And over time, your cells become resistant to insulin's message to soak up glucose, a condition called "insulin resistance." If you develop insulin resistance, your blood sugar remains high, causing damage to your tissues, which then leads to inflammation.

Imbalanced blood sugar levels can be destructive in a few ways. Most crucially, it's thought to reduce the production of reproductive hormones needed to mature your eggs.[655] But also, insulin resistance - a condition when your cells resist the signal from the hormone insulin, caused by elevated levels of insulin by time due to high blood sugar - is associated with oxidative stress, which causes damage to your ovaries. As we learned, oxidative stress also damages the mitochondria needed to provide the energy your eggs need to reach full maturity.[656] And it gets worse. Once your mitochondria get damaged they can further impact insulin resistance.[657] [658]

Insulin and women with PCOS

If you're part of the 15% of women diagnosed with PCOS, this section is especially important for you. For women with PCOS, high insulin levels are known to increase the level of testosterone in the ovaries, which halts the maturation of your eggs. This causes infertility issues related to ovulation, but as it relates to your egg freezing outcome, high blood sugar levels can also cause damage to your eggs by way of oxidative stress.[659] While there are some pharmacological options that can help with managing PCOS, the primary solution lies in your diet. Even more specifically, the solution is managing your blood sugar levels through smart food choices.[660]

Unfortunately, managing your blood sugar is a bit more complex than just eliminating soda or candy. And even if you follow a generally healthy diet, there's a chance your blood sugar levels are still off kilter. In fact, approximately 84 million American adults—more than one out of three—have a condition called pre-diabetes where blood sugar levels are higher than normal, but not high enough to be considered Type 2 diabetes. And, 90% of the people that do have it don't even know it.[661] Part of the reason it's so easy for blood sugars to get out of whack is that managing them properly requires you to think about eating the right foods, in the right format, at the right time and it can be influenced (positively and/or negatively) by other lifestyle factors like stress, sleep and exercise.

Don't get overwhelmed! It's certainly not impossible to regulate your blood sugar levels, it just requires some effort and a bit of a mindshift. And, ideally, no crash dieting, skipping meals or big binges! If you need a little extra motivation to get your blood sugar levels on track, here are a few other peripheral benefits:

- Lower risk of heart disease

- More energy, less fatigue

- More sex drive

- Lowered risk of yeast and bacterial infections

- Less stress (also good for your egg health!)

- Potential weight loss

The key to unlocking these benefits comes from understanding which foods are able to keep your energy levels steady versus those that can take you on a blood sugar roller coaster.

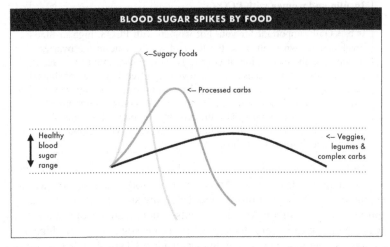

Here's some simple ways to modify your meals to help manage blood sugar:

Look for foods with a low "Glycemic Load" (GL)

Figuring out which foods will inundate your bloodstream with glucose is a bit of a minefield because sugar-laden foods come in a variety of shapes and sizes (even that fancy cold pressed juice can be a wolf in sheep's clothing). You've probably heard about the glycemic index (GI) but have you heard about the glycemic load (GL)? The GI assigns foods a number from 1-100 based on how quickly it will cause a spike in your blood sugar. For example, pure sugar is given a 100 on the GI scale. But what the GI lacks is the ability to tell you how much glucose can be delivered *per serving*. This is where the GL comes in. Many experts believe that it gives you a more holistic picture of the carbs you eat by indicating both how quickly it makes glucose enter the bloodstream and how much glucose per serving it can deliver, when moderated by the other things a food contains, such as fiber.[662] [663]

Carrots are a great example. They have a high GI of 71, so you would think they would cause a massive spike in blood sugar levels. BUT carrots have a low GL of only six, which takes into account the high fiber content that slows down how quickly the sugar hits your bloodstream. That said, if you were to juice a bunch of carrots and take out all the fiber, the glucose doesn't have the fiber to slow its release so it goes straight into your bloodstream.

Low GL: 0 - 10

Moderate GL: 11 - 19
High GL: 20+

Food Guide: Glycemic Load (GL)		
Food	**Serving size**	**Glycemic Load (GL) per serving**
LOW GL (10 or less)		
Asparagus	6 spears	1
Tomatoes	1 cup raw	1
Raw green beans	1/2 cup	1
Raspberries	1 cup	2
Spinach	1 cup steemed	2
Broccoli	1 cup steemed	2
Strawberries	1 cup (sliced)	3
Yogurt plain	8 oz	3
Lentils	1/2 cup cooked	4
Blueberries	1 cup	5
Orange	1 medium	5
Black beans	1/2 cup cooked	5
Apple	1 medium	6
Carrots	1/2 cup	6
Chickpeas	1/2 cup cooked	6
Kidney/pinto beans canned	1/2 cup cooked	6
Beer, Budweiser, 4.9% alcohol	12 oz	7
Sweet corn, from frozen	1/2 cup	7
Grainy bread made with whole seeds and grails	1 slice	7
Wild rice	1/2 cup cooked	7
Oatmeal	1/2 cup cooked	7
Watermelon	1 cup (cubed)	8
Whole wheat pasta	1/2 cup cooked	8
White pasta	1/2 cup cooked	9
Baked beans	1/2 cup cooked	10
White bread	1 slice	10
MODERATE GL (11-19)		
Banana	1 small	11
Orange juice	6 oz	11
Coca-cola	8 oz	13
Cheerios	1 cup	13
Lowfat fruit yogurt	8 oz	14
Sweet potato	1/2 cup mashed	15
White rice	1/2 cup cooked	15
Raisins	1/4 cup	17
Brown rice	1/2 cup cooked	17
Donut	1 medium	17
HIGH GL (20+)		
Corn flakes	1 cup	21
Jelly beans	10 large	22
French fries	1/2 cup	22
Baked potato (Russet)	1 medium	23
Baked potato (white)	1	26
Pancake	6" diameter	39

A downloadable version of this chart is available at
elanzawellness.com.

Find low GL foods full of fiber

In addition to avoiding insulin spikes, low GL foods often come with benefit: fiber. We all keep hearing that we need to eat more fiber, specifically for gut health. But how could it help your reproductive system? Fiber and water work hand-in-hand to assist the body in getting rid of excess hormones and compounds. Fiber is a bit of a sponge. Also, if you don't have enough fiber and water, constipation strikes, which allows for potentially toxic substances (including hormones and carcinogens) to be "re-digested" from fecal matter and returned to the body.[664] Yeah, gross.

EXPERT INSIGHT: "Fiber is incredibly important for feeding our healthy gut bacteria. A healthy gut is crucial for proper macro and micro nutrient absorption, mental health, immunity, and fertility. Nearly every function in the body is impacted if we don't 'feed' our gut bacteria with important nutrients like fiber." - Kaitlyn Noble, Pre and Post-natal Health Coach, Los Angeles

EXPERT INSIGHT: "Fiber is a valuable type of carbohydrate with major benefits that help regulate blood sugars and hunger, as well as prevent constipation." - Elizabeth Stanway-Mayers, Clinical Dietitian, Stanford University Medical Center

On the other hand, don't totally overdo it. Eating an excessive amount of fiber can over-eliminate key hormones needed for quality egg maturation.[665] Considering that only about five percent of Americans meet their recommended daily fiber intake,[666] this is not likely to be an issue but take note if you eat a lot of vegetables, breads or grains. Speaking of carbs...

Don't skip good carbs

It's important to get your energy from all the macronutrient group: this means protein, healthy fats AND carbohydrates. Hating on carbs is second nature to a lot of people, thanks to the myth that carbs of all types are the root cause of weight gain, but dieticians say it's important you eat 45-65% of total calories from carbohydrates. Putting it into context, if you maintain a 2,000 calorie per day diet, the recommended amount of carbohydrate within that would be 225-325gm per day (carbohydrates have four calories per gram). But it's not just about getting a sufficient amount of carbohydrates, it's about getting them from the right sources as well.

EXPERT INSIGHT: "About half of our total calories should come from carbohydrate sources, which serve as fuel for the brain, heart, and lungs. If you have been avoiding carbohydrates, I would recommend starting to get in three to four options of carbohydrates per meal." - Elizabeth Stanway-Mayers, Clinical Dietitian, Stanford University Medical Center

Replace processed carbs with whole ones

Not all carbs are created equal. You might not put carbohydrates like french friends in the same food category as candy but they can affect your blood sugar levels just the same. For example, half a cup of french fries has a GL of 22, which is exactly the same as ten jelly beans. As a rule of thumb, most highly processed or refined carbohydrates such as white bread, white rice and packaged foods can send you on a blood sugar rollercoaster, which can be harmful to your reproductive health. The proverbial proof is in the (sugar-laden) pudding: one study found that women who regularly ate these types of refined carbs were 78% more likely to have ovulatory infertility issues compared to women that incorporated complex carbs from whole grains in their diet.[667]

DOCTOR PERSPECTIVE: "There is resounding evidence regarding processed foods causing dysregulation in blood sugar and therefore destabilizing your mood and stress levels. Clean eating is extremely beneficial in helping stabilize blood glucose which then helps control hormones abating stress and overall improving mood." - Dr. Hemalee Patel, Lifestyle Medicine Expert, San Francisco

Tips for managing your blood sugar:

- Front-load your food intake towards the beginning of the day.[668] Your body becomes more insulin resistant as the day goes on, so a meal you have in the morning is less likely to cause a blood sugar spike than it is in the evening.

- Drink lots of water. It helps your kidneys get rid of excess blood sugar.[669]

- Eat meals at the same time every day to keep blood sugar levels more stable. [670]

- Include lots of low-GL vegetables at each meal. Lightly steam them, or eat them raw.

- Introduce more pulses into your diet (e.g. beans and lentils). They are low GL and count towards your five-a-day, while also serving as good sources of protein.

- Always include protein as part of each meal.

- Snack on dark chocolate or nuts, rather than refined treats.

- Many of the other lifestyle factors we'll be covering in the upcoming chapters will also have a beneficial influence on your blood sugar levels, such as getting quality sleep and engaging in moderate exercise.

EXPERT INSIGHT: "In general, avoid 'naked' carbs – always add on a healthy fat or protein. Starchy vegetables and fruits are significantly better than processed grains thanks to their fiber and nutrient levels, but it's still helpful to add on a small amount of protein/fat for optimal digestion. Plus many of the vitamins found in fruits/veg are fat-soluble, so small amounts of fat will help your body utilize their nutrition more effectively." - Kaitlyn Noble, Pre and Post-natal Health Coach, Los Angeles

8. Be conscious of caffeine

It used to be thought that caffeine had a purely harmful effect on fertility, but as more data from large studies has emerged, conflicting results have made the link less clear - with some showing no negative impact at all.[671 672 673 674]

The key might lie in the *amount* of caffeine consumed. The present thinking is that while low to moderate caffeine consumption has not been shown to have a negative effect on fertility treatments,[675] moderate to high intake could be harmful to your eggs.[676] Support for this comes from studies in which women who consume large amounts of caffeine have been shown to take longer to get pregnant, and exhibit increased rates of miscarriage, spontaneous abortion, fetal death and stillbirth,[677] as well as a decrease in quality embryos.[678] For women who drank four to seven cups of coffee a day, the chance of stillbirth rose by nearly 80%, rising further still to a 300% increased risk for those who drank over eight cups a day.[679 680 681]

The exact biomechanics of caffeine's impact on fertility are still unknown; however, there are a few passageways that can offer us clues. First, caffeine magnifies your body's stress response, raising blood pressure and noradrenaline even at rest, which could have a knock on effect to reproductive hormones.[682 683 684 685 686] Second, when you drink caffeine close to mealtime, it can interfere with your body's ability to absorb key minerals like zinc and iron from your food.[687] [688] It's also theorized that high amounts of caffeine could restrict blood flow to the ovaries and womb, though this could also be due to some other substance present in coffee but not in other caffeine sources such as green tea.[689]

Basically - the jury's out. To be on the safe side, it doesn't hurt to limit your coffee intake. However, if you're as keen on coffee as we are, the good news is that cutting it out completely is not considered mandatory. Instead, doctors commonly advise to limit caffeine consumption to one to two cups per day prior to egg freezing, the same rule of thumb that applies during pregnancy. BUT, let's be clear, this does not mean one to two venti-sized Starbucks coffee cups. The range of safe consumption is considered to be 200mg of caffeine per day.[690] There's quite a considerable range of caffeine per ounce, even from one coffee shop to another, based on the roast they use (dark roast doesn't mean more caffeine than a light roast!) and by the strength at which they brew it. See how your trip to the local coffee shop stacks up:

Caffeine amounts (mg) by brand and size				
SIZE	Starbucks	Dunkin' Donuts	Peet's Coffee	Seattle's Best
Small	155	150	134	125
Medium	235	210	200	166
Large	310	300	267	208
Extra large	410	359	301	N/A

Exact amounts are subject to variation based on brewing strength and style.

EXPERT INSIGHT: "It's important to do a gut check on how caffeine impacts you, regardless of what data suggests. The rush of energy from a morning cup of coffee can be the main motivator for getting out of bed in the morning, and can be so habitually embedded in our days that we never stop to think about how it makes us feel. To do this gut check, I always recommend clients cut out caffeine for a few weeks, then add it back in to increase awareness around its impact. If you notice increased anxiety, irritability, or an energy crash a few hours later, this can be indicative you need to switch to a lower-caffeine or herbal tea. Also, simply having coffee with food or a bit of fat like cream, versus first thing in the morning on an empty stomach, can also impact how you process caffeine." - Kaitlyn Noble, Pre and Post-natal Health Coach, Los Angeles

EXPERT INSIGHT: "Caffeine is dehydrating so it can be counteractive, since hydration is critical in optimizing egg health. If you do drink coffee, be extra diligant about drinking water throughout the day." - Elizabeth Stanway-Mayers, Clinical Dietitian, Stanford University Medical Center

Is decaf coffee ok?

Switching to decaf may present some benefits. But while it contains the beneficial antioxidants of coffee without the problems associated with caffeine and the elevated stress response, decaf coffee is still acidic and may negatively affect your digestive flora. If you're picking out a decaf coffee, look for the Organic Seal, which, as well as the usual pesticides, also prohibits chemical solvents from being used during the caffeine stripping process.

Herbal teas, please

Naturally caffeine-free teas are a great alternative. Even teas with caffeine tend to have less caffeine than coffee, though the amounts do vary. The level depends on how strongly you brew your tea, as well as how caffeinated the tea itself is. In general, white tea has the least caffeine, green tea has a little more caffeine, and black tea has the most. Herbal teas are a smart replacement, as they contain zero caffeine and no problems with acidity.[691] We're big fans of rooibos tea, which is naturally caffeine free and packed with antioxidants.

9. Stick to non-sugary drinks

Considering that caffeine and the insulin spikes from sugar aren't great for your fertility, it should come as no surprise that soda (both diet and regular) and even fruit juices are bad news for your eggs. Research has shown that women who drink one or more sodas per day are 25% less likely to conceive in any given month compared to those that don't.[692] And for women going through IVF, soda has been linked to fewer mature eggs retrieved, lower fertilization rates, and lower quality embryos compared to women who didn't drink them.[693] Artificial sweeteners used in many diet versions have also been associated with higher rates of infertility, but the evidence is not conclusive.[694]

While fruit juices do contain a small amount of vitamins and antioxidants, the overwhelming amounts of sugar could be problematic for egg health. Many fruit juices pack in even more sugar than sodas.[695] The reason fruit juices are so much worse for you than the fruit itself comes down to its high glycemic load (GL). Without any natural fiber to surround the fruit juice, it goes straight into your bloodstream causing a massive insulin spike.

The other issue with sugary beverages is that they might actually make you consume *more* because your body doesn't register drinking calories the same way it does eating them. Drinking doesn't contribute to fullness, though the sugar contributes to caloric intake, which means you're likely to consume more overall and risk getting heavier than the fertility-friendly weight zone (BMI of 20-25).[696]

10. Be alcohol aware

Do you have to give up wine?! This is a big question for a lot of women when they're preparing to freeze their eggs. While the science says drinking alcohol heavily *during* pregnancy is a definite no-no,[697] the evidence linking alcohol to reduced fertility and/or ART outcomes is still considered a matter of debate.

Some studies have associated low to moderate levels of alcohol consumption with decreased fertility, while others have found no association, and some have even found a beneficial association.[698 699 700 701 702 703 704 705 706 707 708 709 710 711 712] The conflicting results from studies are partly due to differences in outcome indicators and study design,[713 714 715] and because of confounding factors like types of drinks consumed,[716 717] lifestyle and age. Drinks may also contain other toxicants or additives and are often consumed alongside other things that might be bad news for your reproductive health such as processed meats.[718] In other words, it's hard to single out one dietary factor from the wider lifestyle of study participants.

Despite the contradictions, the most robust understanding so far comes from a 2017 meta-analysis of 19 different studies measuring the effects of alcohol on the fertility of 98,657 women, which found that light alcohol consumption was associated with an 11% reduction in probability of conceiving, and a 23% reduction in probability of conceiving for moderate-heavy drinking.[719]

When it comes to the impact that alcohol can have on IVF success rates, most studies indicate that alcohol is fine to a point. However, the point at which negative repercussions appear varies from study to study: one study indicates that up to 12 grams of alcohol per day is fine (the standard American drink is 14 grams),[720] and others say that fewer than four drinks per week is ok.[721] [722] Another concluded that women who drank more than seven drinks per week were just two percent less likely to have a live birth per cycle than non-drinkers,[723] so the difference may not be big enough to be significant.

In addition to how much you drink, *when* you drink might also matter. That is, drinking alcohol during the month and week preceding your egg retrieval might have a more negative effect. For example, one study found that risk of IVF failure increased more than four times for women who drank 12 grams of alcohol per day in the week before retrieval and almost three times for those that drank in the month prior. Another study shows that women who consumed one additional drink per day compared to those that had one less drink in the few weeks prior to egg retrieval were slightly more than two times more likely to have a miscarriage, were almost three times less likely to get pregnant, and had a 13% decrease in the number of eggs retrieved during IVF.[724] It's hard to say whether those women who didn't drink were making other, beneficial lifestyle changes too, though, and those who drank had not made any other modifications - which could skew the results.

It's still not completely clear *why* alcohol could harm fertility.[725] One theory is that it affects hormone concentrations. A study found 14 drinks a week, in contrast to no alcohol, is linked to increased estrogen, which could in turn lower FSH and suppress egg development and ovulation.[726] Another theory is that alcohol causes oxidative stress on the ovaries, which could cause harm to your ovaries in the short and long term - potentially exacerbating age-related infertility altogether.[727] [728] In other words, the more alcohol you drink, your shorter your fertile years could be.

While the overarching link between alcohol and reduced fertility is clear,[729] almost every doctor we've spoken to says that having a glass here and there before your egg freezing cycle isn't going to make a drastic impact on your outcome. If you are going to enjoy a bit of alcohol in moderation, red wine could be a better choice as it is host to the antioxidant resveratrol, which is thought to help reduce oxidative stress.[730] [731] It's also best to drink it with a low GL meal in order to prevent insulin spikes.

BONUS SECTION!
11. Bacteria & the vaginal microbiome

What the future may hold for diet and fertility...

There's been an explosion of interest around the concept of gut health and its potential impact on everything from digestion to mental health.[732] [733] So you might have heard of the "gut microbiome" but have you heard of the "vaginal microbiome?" Similar to your gut, your reproductive regions are teaming with thousands of microbes, some good and some bad. While this is an incredibly complex and mutable ecosystem, there is a growing body of evidence that suggests the type and abundance of vaginal and womb microbiomes have the potential to greatly impact your reproductive health.[734]

It helps to think of your vaginal microbiome as a living, evolving ecosystem in which many factors influence the stability of the vaginal microbiota (the ecological community of microorganisms - including good bacteria - that vaginas play host to.) This is because the composition of vaginal communities fluctuate and differ from person to person as a function of age, ethnicity, pregnancy, infections, birth control and sexual behaviors. Even exposure to spermicides or other antimicrobials can decrease the prevalence of the most dominant vaginal bacteria (Lactobacilli for Caucasians, whereas African American women are more likely to have a diverse microbial profile[735]) and consequently increase susceptibility to vaginal infections[736] [737] [738] [739] [740] [741] [742] such as bacterial vaginosis, yeast infections, sexually transmitted infections, urinary tract infections, and HIV.[743] [744] [745] [746] [747] [748] [749] [750] [751] [752]

New research is focusing on the role that vaginal bacteria could play in pregnancy and fertility treatment outcomes, too.[753] Due to the fact that hormones in your body dictate the type of bacteria present within the vaginal microbiome, the hormones administered during the ovarian stimulation phase leading up to your egg retrieval procedure could potentially disrupt the delicate bacterial balance that protects you from disease.[754] [755] [756] In light of this, you might want to be extra vigilant about getting plenty of good bacteria through your diet and/or by taking a probiotic supplement during the hormonal stimulation phase and a week or two after retrieval.[757] [758] Because every vaginal microbiome is unique, it's difficult to "prescribe" a protocol that will help restore a balanced bacterial community. However, scientists have found that the microbiota of healthy premenopausal woman is often dominated by Lactobacillus species, so it could be beneficial to incorporate foods and supplements that are rich in that specific class of probiotics.[759] [760] The good news is that restoring healthy microbes can be done in just a few days.[761]

Lactobacillus boosting foods to support your vaginal microbiome:

- **Yogurt** - Yogurt contains lactobacillus from the cultures added to milk to ferment and thicken the final product.[762] Some yogurts are richer in probiotics than others and many of them are absolute "no no's" because of their high sugar content. The National Yogurt Association (NYA) has created a "live and active cultures" seal in which manufacturers must provide evidence of the bacterial content.

- **Kefir** - Similar to yogurt, kefir is a fermented milk drink made using kefir grains and cow's milk (though it can also be made with goat, sheep and coconut milk or water). The bacteria and yeast ferment lactose (the sugar in milk) into lactic acid, which activates the (good) bacteria to grow.

- **Sauerkraut & kimchi** - Sauerkraut & kimchi are traditionally fermented with naturally occurring bacteria found on cabbage; however, only unpasteurized versions (most likely found in the refrigerated section of the grocery store) contains lactobacillus because the pasteurization process kills the bacteria.

- **Probiotic supplements** - Oral lactobacillus rhamnosus and lactobacillus fermentum supplementation have been shown to restore healthy vaginal flora in up to 82% of women with previous vaginal dysbiosis, specifically an increase in Lactobacillus species.[763] There are even a few vaginal probiotics on the market now that contain a combination of Lactobacillus rhamnosus and Lactobacillus reuteri, which are shown to restore the vaginal microbiome and treat yeast infections as well as bacterial vaginosis.[764] [765]

Key Takeaways

- Switch to a Mediterranean meal mindset, focusing on vegetables, fruit, healthy fats, lean protein, nuts, seeds and whole grains, while avoiding sugars (including artificial sweeteners), simple carbohydrates, fast food, and packaged food. Try to fill half your plate with vegetables and some fruits, and avoid "empty" calories.

- Eat foods closest to their natural form.

- Try to get more of your protein from vegetables and fish, rather than red meat.

- Pick foods with a low glycemic load (GL).

- Limit caffeine consumption, try naturally caffeine free teas.

- Limit alcohol consumption - if you do drink, opt for red wine with a low GL meal.

- Mix up your meals your meals to make them richer in vitamins, minerals and antioxidants for egg health.

- Consider taking a probiotic (namely lactobacillus acidophilus), particularly during the stimulation phase and for a few weeks after your retrieval surgery.

Remember that eating for egg health not only sets you up for your best egg freezing procedure, but is a way of living that will positively influence your reproductive health in general.

EXPERT PERSPECTIVE: "From the new changes you adopt when optimizing your egg health, you're really creating powerful habits that will also impact your nutrition if and when you decide to get pregnant in the future. The quality of your diet is essential for your future baby's health." - Elizabeth Stanway-Mayers, Clinical Dietitian, Stanford University Medical Center

Chapter 9: Supplementing Your Diet

"Success is a science; if you have the conditions, you get the result."

- Oscar Wilde

From "skinny" teas that promise you a flat stomach, to pills that make your hair grow, there are more than 85,000 supplement products (including a huge number for fertility products) for sale in the US market alone.[766][767] Who among us hasn't fallen for the far-fetched claims of at least one "silver bullet?" We're bombarded every time we open Instagram or walk down the pharmacy aisle, so it's never been more important to be a discerning shopper.

Separating the snake oil from the supplements that can deliver real benefit is no easy feat, so this chapter does the heavy lifting and lays out the actual evidence (or warnings about) the major supplements that are implicated in egg quality and fertility. At the end of this chapter, we'll also give you practical tips on how to navigate through the marketing and pick the best brands from the bunch. That way, you and your doctor can make an informed choice on whether or not one or more is right for you.

(Note that this refers to dietary supplements, not prescription or over-the-counter medications.)

Do any supplements actually work?

There *are* certain supplements that have been consistently identified as being helpful for treating infertility and for increasing the success rates of various fertility treatments,[768][769][770] and the science indicates there is an approach to supplements that may have potential benefits for your eggs. However, it's useful to think of them as the icing on top, rather than the whole cake.

Despite the possible benefits the supplements we discuss below can offer, it's important to note that no supplement has been proven beyond all doubt to assist with fertility. Scientists consider *certain* supplements to be "biologically plausible" as fertility enhancers (we'll go into those), but across the board, more well-designed, randomized studies are needed to establish scientific consensus.[771] Until then, they will always be a controversial topic.

Bear in mind that the internet is awash with half-truths and misrepresentations about all kinds of fertility fixes - things that really *won't* work. So, it's smart to stand back and raise your eyebrows every time you hear a new claim about a fertility miracle pill or potion.

Why might my doctor be skeptical of supplements?

Supplements are controversial because of all the unknowns. First, there is not a huge amount of relevant empirical data on whether many supplements actually work or not.[772] Doctors work within the limits set by guidelines published by their professional bodies - before something is adopted as a guideline it has to have reliable data to support it, and many pills and potions lack the robust testing required for doctors to even *consider* recommending them to you. This is because of the loose regulations governing supplements, and the relatively smaller profit margins of supplements compared to patentable drugs - many supplements do not undergo clinical trials on their effects before they are put into bottles and sold.[773]

That's why you might encounter conflicting advice and opinions about what you "should" be taking, or whether you should be taking any supplements at all in the first place. Bear in mind that many doctors are less than enthusiastic about "prescribing" supplements or support their use. This is mostly due to the limited scientific support for many of the wider claims being made by those brands writing a clickbait headline about everything under the sun being "fertility boosting." Your doctor should be the main port of call for your medical care. But our philosophy is that you should be also be armed with the facts and understand what the research scientists are saying, in order to help make up your mind on what is right for you.

Second, supplements have the potential to be risky if improperly taken, and it's your doctor's job to protect you. While supplements can plug holes when it comes to deficiencies, there is the potential for overdosing on certain vitamins and minerals.[774] (Yes, that's an actual thing that we'll cover.)

Finally, in the opinions of some, supplements are a "waste of money" because you should be able to get everything you need from a healthy, balanced diet. In principle, yes, you can. However, there are many caveats to this that make this view too broad-brush and not based in fact, as we'll discover...

If I eat healthily, do I really need to take supplements?

In an ideal world no, but in reality studies suggest that many people - even well fed people in developed countries - aren't getting all the right nutrients from their diets alone[775] [776] and could benefit from dietary supplementation.[777] [778] [779] [780]

It's interesting that we often frame deficiencies as a developing world issue, but micronutrient deficiencies are a genuine phenomenon in parts of the adult population in the US.[781] While the advice is *not* to think of egg freezing as an insurance policy, that *is* exactly how you should think of supplements. Given attaining the "perfect" diet is extremely hard, and different for each person, supplements can function as your fail-safe if your diet isn't quite getting there on its own.

When it comes to enhancing your egg quality, supplements fall into two camps: those that claim to *maintain* a healthy reproductive system by filling dietary gaps, and those that claim to *improve* fertility outcomes, especially when taken in excess of normal dietary quantities. More specifically, one of the central applications of supplements in the context of your egg health is to make sure you are filled with the right nutrients that can protect your eggs from oxidative damage, while simultaneously potentially improving your ovarian function by reducing the likelihood and effects of some conditions that affect it, for example, diabetes.[782]

How likely am I to have a deficiency?

Surprisingly likely, actually. According to the USDA, over 90% of Americans are deficient in one or more vitamins or minerals.[783] It's also important to note that "deficient" just means less than the minimum amount necessary to prevent deficiency-based diseases, not that which is near the levels required for *optimized* health. There are several factors that scientists believe contribute to the US having a sky high deficiency rate, despite being a modern, developed nation. These include the shift in our food systems[784] and lifestyle choices, as well as natural age-related declines:

- *People are heavier on average* - You may have heard the phrase "overfed and undernourished," because the two can easily coexist. One study showed that women with micronutrient deficiencies are over 80% more likely to be obese than non-deficient women.[785]

- *Disordered eating is common* - One in 200 American women suffers from anorexia, while two to three in 100 suffer from bulimia, according to the National Eating Disorder

Association. Restrictive eating and eating disorders in general are linked to nutrient deficiency. If you have a mass index (BMI) under 18.5, you are statistically at risk of being malnourished.[786]

- *An abundance of weight loss / fad diets* - Since their explosion in the eighties, there have been endless variations of restrictive fad diets. One study evaluated four popular diet plans: Atkins for Life diet (similar to the keto diet), The South Beach Diet, the DASH diet, and the Best Life diet, to see if they hit the government's minimum micronutrient recommendations. The researchers found that vitamin B7, vitamin D, vitamin E, chromium, iodine and molybdenum were consistently low or nonexistent in all four diet plans.[787] Remember, anytime you limit or cut out an entire macronutrient group (carbohydrates, fat, or animal products) through extreme eating, you risk missing important nutrients.

- *Celiac disease & other malabsorptive disorders* - One study showed that 20–38% of celiac patients experience nutritional deficiencies that include proteins, dietary fiber, minerals, and vitamins.[788] [789] People with digestive system conditions like Crohn's disease are often considered at higher risk of malnourishment.[790] [791]

- *Vegans and vegetarians* - Studies have shown low dietary intake of vitamin B12 and D, calcium, and omega-3 fatty acids, iron and zinc in strict vegetarians.[792] [793] [794]

- *Eating intensively farmed foods* - Overuse of pesticides can cause soil to degrade over time, as populations decline of beneficial soil microorganisms (like fungi and bacteria) that are useful to plant growth. A study reviewed the US Department of Agriculture nutritional data from both 1950 and 1999 for 43 different vegetables and fruits, finding "reliable declines" in the amount of protein, calcium, phosphorus, iron, riboflavin (vitamin B2) and vitamin C over the past half century. The researchers believe the declining nutritional content is due to modern agricultural practices which are designed to improve marketable traits like size, growth rate, and pest resistance, to the detriment of nutrition.[795] In effect, a carrot now may not have the same nutritional profile now as a carrot did in 1950. Soil scientists liken the degradation of soil through overuse to the overuse of antibiotics.

- **Smoking** - Smoking can interfere with the absorption of nutrients from foods.[796]

- **Taking birth control pills** - Oral contraceptives are known to play a role in nutrient deficiencies, possibly affecting absorption.[797] Studies have shown that they are linked to deficiencies in the following:[798] folic acid,[799] [800] vitamins B2, B6, B12,[801] [802] vitamin C,[803] vitamin E,[804] [805] magnesium,[806] [807] selenium,[808] zinc,[809] and phosphorus.[810]

Even if you are more at risk of nutrient deficiencies, be aware that some supplements may not be suitable for you. Always check with your doctor about adverse side effects or risks before taking any supplements. In addition to the supplements we'll cover below, if you have a specific health condition your doctor may recommend additional supplements, which for example could include iron supplements if blood tests show you are anemic (iron deficient).

Also bear in mind that a specific supplement regime has not been established for ovarian stimulation cycles (before IVF or egg freezing). That's why you might see some dosages referred to in this section as "for pregnant women" as it is the best possible proxy for egg health.

Navigating the supplements section

After reading this next chapter, you should feel more clear and confident knowing how to best tackle that overcrowded drugstore aisle. After weighing up the data and the drama around supplements, here's what we think are the key supplements for fertility:

Multivitamin and mineral supplements
Folic Acid
Vitamin B12
Zinc
Selenium
Iodine

Stand-alone supplements
Coenzyme Q10 (Ubiquinol)
Omega 3 Fatty Acids (EPA & DHA)
Melatonin

Supplements for women with PCOS
Myo-inositol
Myo-inositol + alpha-lipoic acid

Supplements for women with a diminished ovarian reserve
DHEA

The jury's out on these supplements tied to fertility
L-arginine
Vitamin D
Vitamin E
Vitamin C
Iron
Resveratrol
Catechins (+Quercetin/OPC)
Diosgenin
Pycnogenol
Maca
Chinese herbs

Supplements to *avoid* for egg freezing
Royal Jelly
Chasteberry (chastetree, chaste tree berry, Vitex, monk's pepper, lilac chastetree)
St. John's Wort

Then, when you're ready to hit the pharmacy aisle... HOW TO: Buying the best brands and bottles

Multivitamin and mineral supplements

Taking a daily prenatal multivitamin is an easy way to get a lot of nutrients in one pill, many of which help the absorption of others in the mix. It's kind of strange to see a bottle of prenatal *anything* on your bathroom shelf (and a good way to give a partner a shock), but it is what it is!

Most prenatal supplements are blended for the needs of women who are already pregnant, but they also contain valuable vitamins and antioxidants that can enhance and protect your eggs during maturation. Increasingly, preconception formulations are hitting the shelves, too, as companies try to innovate; more on that later when we get into picking the right brand.

The downside of all-in-one prenatal supplements is that few of them supply all the desired vitamins/antioxidants in the precise amounts that are most beneficial to your eggs, as outlined below. If you find a prenatal vitamin that you like, but it doesn't have sufficient amounts of one or more key nutrients, you might want to "top up" with a separate supplement specifically of that nutrient. That's why we also cover stand-alone supplements. *Do not* simply take more than the daily dosage of the prenatal, because you could risk an overdose of other vitamins also included in the supplement. In particular, be aware that vitamin A - which is often found in multivitamins and prenatals - can be harmful if you take more than 10,000 international units (IU) on a daily basis.[811]

There are usually a lot of different vitamins and minerals included in a prenatal supplement, many of which could play a role in optimizing reproductive health. But, below is our evidence-based "Big Five" of the vitamins and minerals normally found in prenatal supplements, which research has shown can improve or protect your eggs, whether directly or indirectly:

Check that your prenatal includes the following "The Big Five" at adequate levels:

1. Folic Acid (also called folate or vitamin B9)

First up, let's look at the famous "pregnancy supplement;" you may have already heard of this vitamin, its links with healthy conception and pregnancy and it's ability to prevent birth defects. In particular, folic acid is thought to reduce the chance of babies developing with neural tube defects that can affect their brains and spinal cords and result in conditions like spina bifida. The research is so compelling that the Centers for Disease Control and Prevention (CDC) recommends that all women of reproductive age take 400 mcg supplement even if they are not planning a pregnancy because many of these defects form before women usually even know they're pregnant.[812]

In addition, studies on folic acid supplementation has shown it to help:

- Lower the frequency of infertility[813]

- Lower the risk of miscarriage[814]

- Confer greater success in infertility treatment.[815]

- Increase the number of eggs retrieved[816]

- Improve the maturation and quality of eggs[817 818 819 820]

- Counter free radicals and reduce oxidative stress[821]

Although most Americans consume adequate amounts of folate in their diets (it is added to all flour during manufacturing), taking a folic acid supplement is often recommended because, ironically, women of childbearing age are more at risk of insufficient folate intakes than other people.[822] Even when intakes of folic acid from dietary supplements are included, 17% of women aged 19 to 30 years do not get the daily requirement.[823]

While the folate found in foods is better absorbed than synthetic versions, it is a water-soluble vitamin, so the body cannot store it, which is another reason most doctors recommend daily supplementation.[824]

You might be particularly susceptible to a folic acid deficiency if... you're a smoker or a heavy drinker (more motivation to cut down or cut them out!).[825] [826] If you've been taking birth control pills, they can interfere with your body's ability to metabolize folate. And if you have a malabsorptive disorder, such as celiac disease or inflammatory bowel disease, you might be absorbing less folate than other people, even if you eat lots of folate-rich foods such as leafy greens, legumes and eggs.[827]

About 40% to 60% of people have a genetic variation whereby they cannot complete the final step of converting folic acid in the body to the active form, l-methylfolate/5-MTHF. So even if these people have a diet rich in legumes, broccoli and green leafy vegetables they could still have a deficiency that can lead to a build-up of homocysteine.[828] [829] Certain medications, such as anti-seizure drugs, could also lead to a 5-MTHF deficiency.

Symptoms of folate deficiency can include: weakness, fatigue, difficulty concentrating, irritability, headache, heart palpitations, and shortness of breath.[830]

Safety and side effects:

Folic acid is considered to be non-toxic, even at high doses. However, you should not take more than 1000mcg per day unless under the advice of your doctor.[831] [832]

You might come across scary stories online about folate intake being linked to colorectal cancer. However, a study in the respected Lancet journal looked at data from 50,000 people and found no significant differences in those taking folic acid. Something you *should* be aware of, though, is that high doses of folic acid can mask symptoms of B12 deficiency.[833]

Recommended dosage:

If you are taking folic acid, a minimum of 400 to 800 mcg per day is usually suggested[834] (ideally 600 mcg[835]) as part of a prenatal vitamin or in a separate supplement.

When/how to take it:

Try to take your folic acid supplement without food, as then it is nearly 100% bioavailable (vs. only 85% if taken with food).[836][837]

2. Vitamin B12

B12 is an essential vitamin that your body can't make from other things - i.e. you can only get B12 through diet and supplements. It is a necessary cofactor for DNA synthesis, a crucial activity that occurs during egg maturation. Nearly nine percent of US adults absorb too little B12 through their diets and nearly 39% are considered in the "low" range.[838][839][840] As well as being a concern for general health, B12 deficiencies have implications for fertility. Women with vitamin B12 deficiencies undergoing IVF are more likely to have fewer eggs retrieved, lower quality eggs and lower quality embryos.[841][842]

You might be particularly susceptible to a B12 deficiency if... you regularly take antacids, if you have been diagnosed with pernicious anemia (which is more likely if someone else in your family had it or has it, or if you are of Northern European or Scandinavian descent), if you have had gastrointestinal surgery, such as weight loss surgery, or if you have a digestive disorder, such as celiac disease or Crohn's disease. These conditions can decrease the amount of vitamin B12 that the body can absorb.[843]

Because only foods derived from animals have naturally occurring vitamin B12, vegetarians and vegans are thought to be particularly susceptible to deficiencies.[844][845][846] However, a study of almost 4,000 people curiously found no difference in the B12 levels of those ate meat and those who did not.[847] Interestingly, the results even suggested that fortified cereals, dairy products and dietary supplementation, if anything, provide *better* protection against B12 deficiency than relying on B12 from meat consumption. Vegans and vegetarians who are vigilant may be protecting themselves better against deficiency, given the well-publicized risk. Lastly, small studies and case reports suggest that 10%–30% of patients who take metformin (a medicine usually used to treat type 2 diabetes) have reduced vitamin B12 absorption.[848][849]

Signs of vitamin B12 deficiency include: fatigue, weakness, constipation, loss of appetite, and weight loss, difficulty maintaining balance, depression, confusion, personality changes, dementia, poor memory, and soreness of the mouth or tongue. Neurological changes, such as numbness and tingling in the hands and feet, can also occur.[850] It just takes a simple blood test to check your B12 level to see if you have a deficiency.

What to buy:

In dietary supplements, vitamin B12 is often labeled as cyanocobalamin or methylcobalamin.[851] Existing evidence does not suggest any differences among forms with respect to absorption or bioavailability.[852] You might also come across tablets or lozenges that claim to have higher bioavailability, but the evidence so far doesn't support these claims.[853] [854]

Vegans and vegetarians may prefer to supplement their diet using nutritional yeast, rather than standard supplements, which are often animal-derived. Nutritional yeast (often called "nooch" for shorthand!) is an inactive form of yeast made from a single-celled organism, which is grown on molasses. That means no animals are involved in making it, because yeasts are members of the fungi family, like mushrooms. If it's not stocked at your grocery store, check your local natural food store. Check the label, as not all brands of nooch contain B12.

Safety and side effects:

According to the American Institute of Medicine (IOM), "no adverse effects have been associated with excess vitamin B12 intake from food and supplements in healthy individuals."[855]

Recommended dosage:

2.6mcg of Vitamin B12 per day.[856]

When/how to take it:

Ideally you can find this as part of a prenatal vitamin, but it can also be found in B-Vitamin complex supplements. Try to take vitamin B12 supplements on an empty stomach when you first wake up in the morning.

3. Zinc

Zinc has shown to be *crucial* to a smooth-running egg maturation process during the 90 days before your egg freezing procedure.[857] [858] [859] [860] [861] [862] [863] [864] [865] [866] [867] [868] Scientists believe that zinc deficiency can negatively affect the early stages of egg development by reducing the ability of the egg cells to divide and be fertilized in the future.[869] One study found that eggs with deficient levels of zinc were "stuck" at the very beginning stages of maturation. But when researchers added zinc to the eggs (in a petri dish), the proper progression of maturation was restored.[870]

If you're interested in the science about zinc

Human eggs contain zinc transporters and zinc vesicles,[871] [872] [873] which require a substantial 50% increase in total zinc content in order to progress through stages of meiosis (chromosomal processing) to reach full maturity. While scientists don't know exactly why zinc is so important, they do know that the flood of it (coined the "zinc flood") to eggs acts as an activator for them to mature.[874] In fact, an exciting new study at Northwestern University indicates that zinc dynamics in an egg could potentially predict whether or not it is good enough quality to develop into an embryo.[875] This means that perhaps one day we'll be able to use zinc to test the quality of eggs retrieved before they are frozen!

You might be particularly susceptible to a zinc deficiency if... you have irritable bowel syndrome, Crohn's disease, sickle cell disease, gastrointestinal disorders or liver disease. Additionally, because the most potent forms of zinc come from meat, vegetarians should be particularly aware of zinc deficiency. This is furthered by the fact that a vegetarian diet typically contains high levels of legumes and whole grains, which contain phytates that bind zinc and inhibit its absorption.[876] [877]

Consuming a lot of calcium or calcium-fortified foods may also reduce both iron and zinc absorption.[878] [879] [880] [881] Something to take note of if you hit those lattes hard. Signs of a deficiency include diarrhea, hair loss, ulcers, stunted growth, poor immune system, lethargy, weight loss, poor wound healing and other skin problems. It is hard to actually measure zinc deficiency using laboratory tests, unfortunately, because of the way it is distributed throughout the body.[882] [883] [884] [885]

What to buy:

Dietary supplements can have several different forms of zinc including zinc gluconate, zinc sulfate and zinc acetate. It is not clear whether one form is better than the others.[886]

Safety and side effects:

Getting *too much* zinc can be harmful. The National Institutes of Health, Office of Dietary Supplements (NIH) states that you should not exceed 40 mg of zinc per day.[887] This is due to some concern that taking doses higher than 40 mg daily might decrease how much copper the body absorbs.[888] This harks back to what we were saying about vitamins and minerals not being lone wolves, but interacting in pairs or as a pack. Signs of too much zinc include nausea, vomiting, loss of appetite, stomach cramps, diarrhea, and headaches.

Recommended dosage:

8mg of zinc per day in supplement form, assuming you are getting a sufficient amount of zinc from your diet. Vegetarians: increase by 50% to 12mg zinc supplement intake per day.[889]

When/how to take it:
Zinc is often included as part of a prenatal vitamin along with copper, which helps decrease the chances of copper malabsorption.

4. Selenium

Interest in selenium has been growing in the past few decades due to its potential to impact multiple areas of human health. Selenium is an essential mineral and antioxidant naturally found in soil, water, and sometimes in food.[890] It is thought to play a role in follicle growth and maturation,[891 892] egg development,[893] as well as the prevention of chromosome breakage due to oxidative stress.[894 895 896]

Two recent studies showed that selenium supplementation could improve the outcome of IVF,[897 898] though both of these studies only involved a small number of women and supplementation was given in combination with other micronutrients. As such, the direct link is not yet proven.[899 900 901]

That said, it is an area of scientific interest given that selenium is found within the follicular fluid that nourishes your eggs.[902] One study found that women with "unexplained" infertility had significantly reduced selenium levels in both follicular fluid and blood.[903]

In animal studies (cows, mice, rats, goats), large, healthy follicles were shown to have ten times the amount of selenium than small or dying follicles.[904] In these animals, selenium has also been shown to improve egg growth,[905 906] repress follicle death,[907] enhance the rate of folliculogenesis, increase production of the hormone estradiol[908] and to reduce the amount of oxidative stress.[909] Pre-conception selenium supplementation in mice was also shown to yield a high occurrence of good quality embryos.[910]

Selenium deficiency, on the other hand, has been shown to cause reproductive and pregnancy complications,[911 912 913 914] ovarian degeneration and follicle death[915] in human and animal studies.

You might be particularly susceptible to a deficiency if... In the US, selenium deficiency is rare,[916] though an estimated one billion people around the world are affected by selenium deficiency.[917] It is generally recognized that selenium intakes across Europe are low, reflecting inadequate soil levels.[918] This is in contrast to the United States, where soil selenium levels tend to be high to adequate.[919 920] A National Diet and Nutrition study in the UK found that 50% of adult women had intakes below recommendations.[921] People in the Middle East and Turkey also often have lower than recommended intakes. Women with endometriosis and PCOS may have lower selenium levels.[922] [923]

Signs of a selenium deficiency can include: hair loss and skin and fingernail discoloration, fatigue, brain fog and difficulty concentrating, Chronic deficiency can lead to hypothyroidism.

What to buy:
Selenium is often included as part of a prenatal supplement but can also be purchased by itself.

Safety and side effects:
There are potential health risks for taking selenium in excess.[924] Acute selenium toxicity can cause severe gastrointestinal and neurological symptoms, acute respiratory distress syndrome, myocardial infarction, hair loss, muscle tenderness, tremors, lightheadedness, facial flushing, kidney failure, cardiac failure, and, in very rare cases, death.[925] [926]

Consuming more than 400mcg of selenium per day is not advised, as it is a trace mineral that can accumulate within the body.[927]

Recommended dosage:
The US Institute of Medicine recommends 60mcg of selenium supplementation per day for pregnant women.[928]

5. Iodine

Iodine is increasingly being linked to sound reproductive health. Researchers have found that women with iodine deficiencies are 46% less likely to conceive compared to women with healthy iodine levels.[929] And for pregnant women, moderate-to-severe iodine deficiency increases the rate of spontaneous abortion and infant mortality.[930] Even mild iodine deficiency during pregnancy may be linked to low intelligence in children. While these studies aren't directly related to egg quality, we do know that iodine is an essential component of thyroid hormones,[931] which themselves are involved in all aspects of reproduction and the delicate balance within the endocrine system. When iodine requirements are not met, the thyroid may no longer be able to synthesize sufficient amounts of thyroid hormone. While most issues are related to fetal development and miscarriage, thyroid function is also implicated in ovulatory disorders.[932] [933]

You might be particularly susceptible to an iodine deficiency if...
Iodine deficiency is considered a global public health problem affecting around 2.2 billion people.[934] Deficiency in the US is not known to be widespread, with iodine naturally present in foods like seaweed, dairy, grains and eggs[935] [936] and added to others, namely salt.[937] However, mild iodine deficiency has reemerged in particular demographics, including women of childbearing age.[938] [939] [940] [941] You should be particularly aware if

you don't consume dairy products,[942] you restrict your salt intake, or you purchase non-iodized salt.[943] If your iodine intake falls below approximately 10–20 mcg per day, hypothyroidism occurs. A goiter (lump on the throat) is usually the earliest clinical sign of iodine deficiency, as low iodine levels can cause an underactive thyroid.[944]

What to buy:

Most prenatal vitamins contain iodine.

Safety and side effects:

According to the American Food and Nutrition Board, you should not exceed 1,100 mcg of iodine per day. (In most people, iodine ingested from foods and supplements are unlikely to exceed this). Some people, such as those with autoimmune thyroid disease, may experience adverse effects with iodine (check with your doctor), but it is considered safe for the general population.[945] [946]

Recommended dosage:

The World Health Organization (WHO) recommends that pregnant women get a total of 250 mcg of iodine per day,[947] [948] though if you get plenty of iodine in your diet, make this 150 mcg in supplement form.

Additional stand-alone supplements

While the above "Big Five" can usually be found in a good quality prenatal multivitamin (more on how to pick that later), there are some other potentially potent players you might want to consider adding in as stand-alone supplements. It's annoying to buy and have to swallow extra pills, but take a look at the evidence and decide for yourself if the negatives are outweighed by the possible upsides:

Coenzyme Q10 (Ubiquinol)

If there's one supplement that might, just might, deserve the title of "super," it's Coenzyme Q10. Also known as CoQ10, this is a powerful antioxidant[949] that shows promise as a supplement to improve egg quality and quantity. CoQ10, among other cofactors, is "a potent stimulator of mitochondrial function,"[950] which basically means that it might help to synthesize energy (ATP) in your cells, including in your ovaries. And, as we learned, egg maturation is a very energy intensive process. Older, worn out mitochondria cannot generally do it as efficiently as younger mitochondria, so if your mitochondria are given a boost, it's a little like rolling the clock back. Simultaneously, CoQ10, as an antioxidant, provides protection against accumulating oxidative stress.[951] [952] [953] [954] [955] [956] Our bodies can also actually produce CoQ10, but this ability declines with age.

In both humans and mice, age-related fertility decline has been linked to decreased expression of enzymes responsible for the production of CoQ10. In mice with depleted ovarian reserves, CoQ10 supplementation was associated with a higher number of eggs, better development of those eggs, and more live births.[957] There has only been one human study, however. And while it showed women age 35-43 years old undergoing IVF who received 600mg supplementation of CoQ10 had improved pregnancy rates and better quality eggs than those who were not supplemented, not enough women were enrolled in the study for the results to be statistically significant,[958] which is why we're talking in terms of "might" and "could."

While it's not fully understood how far CoQ10 can effectively turn back the hands of time yet, and randomized clinical trials in humans are still needed, it does provide promise. Researchers from around the world have stated "it seems clear that supplementation with CoQ10 improves mitochondrial function and confers antioxidant protection for organs and tissues."[959]

The reason CoQ10 is frequently taken as a supplement is because it is found in only very small amounts in foods, including organ meats, fatty fish, spinach, cauliflower, broccoli, oranges, strawberries, lentils and peanuts. Even consuming large amounts of these foods won't provide much of a boost.

Coenzyme Q10 might be particularly beneficial if... you are older than 35 or have low ovarian reserve.[960]

What to buy:

Make sure to buy a supplement labeled "ubiquinol" rather than "ubiquinone." Ubiquinol is a slightly more expensive, active form that is more easily absorbed by the body (some people, particularly people with Hispanic and Chinese heritage, lack the enzyme that converts CoQ10 to ubiquinol). If the label just states CoQ10 without additional information then you can assume it's not the one you want. The label should state "ubiquinol," or "active antioxidant form" or "reduced form."

Safety and side effects:

No safety concerns have been reported, even in very high doses.[961] The only noted side effect has been mild gastrointestinal symptoms in some people.[962] Use is widespread. Many people around the world, including professional athletes, take CoQ10 supplements for their supposed anti-aging and energy metabolism benefits.[963]

Recommended dosage:

It's best to discuss with your fertility doctor but one study indicates that 100mg-600mg of CoQ10 per day can boost fertility.[964] Some doctors on our panel recommend taking 100mg of Ubiquinol three times per day.

When/how to take it:

It's important to note that CoQ10 takes a few weeks or more to build up in tissues, which means that you need to start taking it at least four months prior to your retrieval procedure in order to get the maximum benefit. This will allow the molecule to potentially support your mitochondria during the three months while your eggs are maturing. CoQ10 is best absorbed with a meal, preferably breakfast.

EXPERT INSIGHT: "CoQ10 is a fat-soluble compound, so it's best taken with some fat or oils, such as avocado or yogurt." - Elizabeth Stanway-Mayers, Clinical Dietitian, Stanford University Medical Center

Omega-3 fatty acids (EPA & DHA)

As we reviewed in the "Eating for Egg Health" chapter, a diet high in omega-3 and not too much omega-6 is important for maturing quality eggs - so we can all enjoy tucking into a delicious Mediterranean diet knowing it's doing our eggs good. Omega-3 fatty acids can only be absorbed through food and supplementation.[965] And while omega-6 is plentiful in the Western diet, omega 3 (found in oily fish, seeds, seaweed and walnuts) is not generally consumed in a healthy ratio. This is where supplementation can prove to be useful. Omega-3s are important enough to merit a fail-safe.

While omega-3 from fatty fish is absorbed twice as effectively as even the most potent fish oil supplement,[966] [967] it can be beneficial to take it in supplement form if you dislike these foods or find them challenging to incorporate in the right quantities into your diet.

You might be particularly susceptible to a deficiency if...you don't eat a lot of fatty fish or other omega-3 rich foods. Vegan and vegetarian diets are at a particular risk of having omega-3 deficiency because the main source of omega-3 from plant sources is a type known as ALA, which is poorly absorbed into the body.[968] A deficiency of essential fatty acids can cause rough, scaly skin and dermatitis.[969] You can take a blood test to see if you have the correct levels and ratios of omega-3 to 6.

What to buy:

There are hundreds of different omega-3 supplements on the market, and not all of them are created equal. Formulations vary widely,[970] so it is important to check product labels to determine the types and amounts of omega-3s in these products.

Omega-3 supplements are perishable. When they go rancid, they become less potent and even harmful. Make sure to double check the expiration date before buying, check if the formulation includes an antioxidant like vitamin E (which might help with the lifespan) and avoid buying them in bulk.

Buy supplements with EPA & DHA - There are three main types of fatty acids. EPA (eicosapentaenoic acid), DHA (docosahexaenoic acid), both commonly found in marine oils. ALA (alpha-linolenic acid) is found in plant oils.[971] Research indicates that the two most beneficial and active forms are EPA and DHA. ALA is considered much less effective because your body has to convert ALA into its more active forms, EPA and DHA, and can only do this in small amounts.[972] Vegetarian supplements are available, but they usually only contain ALA. One exception to this is algal oil, which is an excellent source of quality omega-3s and suitable for everyone, including vegans.[973]

Check the amount of EPA & DHA - A supplement may say on the front that it contains 1000 mg fish oil per capsule but only about a third to a half of the oil is actually EPA and DHA. The rest is often other fatty acids that can help with absorption.[974]

Safety and side effects:

According to the European Food Safety Authority, long-term consumption of EPA and DHA supplements at combined doses of up to about 5000 mg/day appears to be safe.[975] The FDA recommends not exceeding 3000 mg/day EPA and DHA combined, with up to 2000 mg/day from dietary supplements.[976] Although seafood contains varying levels of mercury, omega-3 supplements have not been found to contain this contaminant because it is removed during processing and purification.[977] [978] Commonly reported side effects of omega-3 supplements are usually mild. These include unpleasant taste, bad breath, heartburn, nausea, gastrointestinal discomfort, diarrhea, headache, and odoriferous sweat.[979]

Recommended dosage:

According to the National Academy of Medicine, an adequate intake of omega-3s for pregnant women is 1400 mg per day. Check how much you're getting in your diet, then you can supplement with the right amount of fish oil. A three ounce serving of wild-caught salmon, for instance, contains roughly 1830 mg of EPA and DHA.[980]

When/how to take it:

Try to take your fish oil supplement with a meal that contains fat, as fat increases absorption of omega-3s.[981] [982]

Melatonin

Melatonin is a hormone that is secreted at night, indicating to your body that it's time to rest, which is why it's sometimes called "the sleepy hormone."[983] [984] A substantial body of research has shown that this hormone has many functions other than just sleep, many of which pose potential benefits to fertility. For example, it serves as an antioxidant, an anti-inflammatory, an immune modulator,[985] and helps regulate fat and glucose metabolism.[986]

Recent studies have revealed that taking melatonin supplements can restore antioxidant defenses around your eggs, protecting them from oxidative stress that can damage them during maturation.[987] Melatonin's antioxidant properties have been found to be more powerful than those of vitamin C or vitamin E.[988]

One indication comes from studies in which melatonin appears to accumulate preferentially in ovaries compared with other organs[989] and that higher concentrations of melatonin are found in follicular fluid surrounding your eggs.[990] [991] [992] Another study found that larger, more mature follicles in women's ovaries had higher concentrations of melatonin than the smaller ones.[993] Similarly, a study in which women who took a daily melatonin supplement prior to egg retrieval in IVF had an increased proportion of mature eggs and high-quality embryos.[994] (Note that in the study melatonin was taken in conjunction with some other supplements, so it is hard to separate out the precise benefactor).

Even from a long-term standpoint, melatonin seems to provide some benefits to your reproductive health. The researchers from a study conducted on mice that were given melatonin supplements coined it an "anti-aging agent" for the protective benefits they found it to confer on the ovaries.[995]

You might be particularly susceptible to a deficiency if...

Melatonin levels decline with age, which is why it can be particularly beneficial if you are 30+.[996]

What to buy:

Studies have shown that there is a significant amount of variability in the actual melatonin content sold in supplements, which can range from 83% to +478% from the amount listed on the label.[997] Therefore, it's best to buy from well known, high quality brands that have been evaluated by a third party.

Safety and side effects:

According to the US National Center for Complementary and Integrative Health (NCCIH) melatonin "appears to be safe when used short-term, but the lack of long-term studies means we don't know if it's safe for extended use." Side effects of melatonin are uncommon but can include drowsiness, headache, dizziness, or nausea.

It's important to note (potentially for the future) that taking melatonin supplements, especially in combination with progesterone, can potentially disrupt ovulation and as such, should not be taken by women who are trying to conceive naturally.[998] Interestingly, some researchers believe that this is a cue from our evolutionary past in which our bodies suppress ovulation during darker months (a signal communicated by the abundance of melatonin) to prevent babies being born when resources are less abundant.[999]

Additionally, melatonin could interact with certain medications, including antidepressants, blood thinners and blood pressure medications.[1000] [1001] [1002] Always discuss usage with your doctor.

Recommended dosage:

The dose of melatonin used in previous clinical studies on egg quality is a 3mg tablet taken shortly before bed. A "more is more" approach does not work with melatonin; the effect is that of a U shaped curve.

When/how to take it:

It's best to take melatonin in the evening at the same time every day since it affects your sleep-wake cycle and it could cause daytime drowsiness.[1003]

Supplementation for women diagnosed with polycystic ovarian syndrome (PCOS)

If you've been diagnosed with PCOS, you're likely to have insulin resistance, oxidative stress and hormonal imbalances that are most well-known for causing ovulatory issues.[1004] Some studies have also found that women with PCOS tend to retrieve poorer quality eggs,[1005] a trend that is particularly apparent for women with PCOS who are overweight.[1006]

In contrast to women considered "poor responders" to the hormone injections, women with PCOS tend to be hyper responsive.[1007] This means that you probably won't need as much medication as other women but it does put you at higher risk of developing ovarian hyperstimulation syndrome (OHSS).[1008] Lifestyle modifications such as diet and exercise are the paramount for the treatment of PCOS;[1009] however, there is a small but growing amount of research on supplements that could help further benefit your reproductive health. Just like all other supplements, make sure to check with your doctor before taking them.

Myo-inositol for PCOS

Current status: Good evidence but check with your doctor before taking

Myo-inositol is an insulin sensitizer, which is why it's been studied for women with PCOS. While more studies are needed, the majority of the research indicates that supplementing with myo-inositol for a few months prior to fertility treatment can increase the number of mature eggs retrieved, increase overall egg quality, and reduce the risk of OHSS during ovarian stimulation for women with PCOS, especially when supplemented alongside folic acid and alpha-lipoic acid.[1010] [1011] [1012] [1013]

For example, one study showed that overweight women with PCOS who took myo-inositol and folic acid supplements during their IVF cycles had a 32% chance of a successful pregnancy versus just a 12% chance for women who only took a straight folic acid supplement, without the inositol.[1014] Similarly, another study showed that women with PCOS who took myo-inositol for three months before their ART procedure saw a 50% increase in pregnancy rate.[1015]

According to scientists, "Myo-inositol has proven to be a new treatment option for patients with PCOS and infertility. The achieved pregnancy rates are at least in an equivalent or even superior range than those reported using metformin as an insulin sensitizer. No moderate to severe side effects were observed when myo-inositol was used at a dosage of 4000 mg per day. In addition, our evidence suggests that a myo-inositol therapy in women with PCOS results in better fertilization rates and a clear trend to a better embryo quality."[1016]

Myo-inositol + alpha-lipoic acid

Current status: Unproven

When myo-inositol is supplemented with alpha-lipoic acid, preliminary evidence indicates that could have an even more potent effect on increasing insulin sensitivity. One study found that the combined effect helped improve the reproductive outcome of women with PCOS going through IVF, showing a reduction in BMI, insulin levels and an increase in high quality embryos.[1017] Another study on the combined effects of alpha-lipoic acid and myo-inositol found that women with PCOS were able to restore a normal menstrual pattern and hormonal balance.[1018]

Supplementation for women diagnosed with a diminished ovarian reserve

If you've been diagnosed with a diminished ovarian reserve or if you've undergone a previous egg freezing cycle that resulted in very few eggs retrieved, you're likely to have the exact opposite problem as women with PCOS. In this case, your ovaries might not be very responsive to the hormones, which often results in fewer eggs retrieved and eventually lower live birth rates.[1019] In all cases, it is recommended that you speak to your doctor prior to adding supplements to your regime.

DHEA (Dehydroepiandrosterone)

Current status: Good evidence, but possible side effects and not suitable for everyone. Discuss with your doctor.

If testing suggests you may have a diminished ovarian reserve, your doctor might recommend that you take a DHEA supplement for a few months prior to your treatment. It's thought this hormone could give older women, or those with low ovarian reserve, a chance to improve both the quality and quantity of the eggs retrieved in the procedure.[1020] [1021] DHEA is a hormone that's naturally produced in your adrenal gland and ovaries. It's known to contribute to various aspects of reproduction, and because it can decrease by up to 80% throughout adulthood,[1022] scientists believe that supplementing with DHEA could enable the ovaries to function more like that of a younger woman.[1023]

That said, many doctors are concerned about the potential risks of taking a steroid hormone, especially when the benefits are not yet proven. Nevertheless, a growing body of evidence does support the notion that DHEA is a potentially useful supplement.[1024] Initial research supports the hypothesis that supplementing with DHEA can increase the quantity of eggs retrieved by either increasing the pool of follicles that are recruited into the beginning stages of maturation and/or increasing the proportion of eggs that survive the beginning stages of maturation without dying off.[1025] [1026] [1027] DHEA supplements are also thought to increase the quality of eggs by recreating the environment in which the eggs mature to match that of a younger woman, which allows the eggs to process chromosomes correctly.[1028] [1029]

Research is inconsistent and patchy, and more studies are needed to confirm its effectiveness and safety,[1030] so the takeaway is that DHEA is definitely something to talk to your doctor about, rather than considering going it alone.

DOCTOR PERSPECTIVE: "Our patients with diminished ovarian reserve supplement with DHEA for at least 6-8 weeks before their IVF cycle starts. DHEA supplementation has been one of the major drivers of our patients' success - including the almost 48-year-old patient who had a daughter with her own eggs after IVF following DHEA supplementation. Using DHEA is a much more physiological approach than using testosterone directly. When DHEA is converted into testosterone in the body, each organ, ovaries included, takes in as much testosterone as it needs, keeping side effects to a minimum." - Dr. Norbert Gleicher, Center for Human Reproduction, New York City

DOCTOR PERSPECTIVE: "Many of my patients complain about the side effects of DHEA - so I think they are worth mentioning. Because it is an androgen (male hormone), it can cause acne and facial hair. It can also cause fatigue and GI issues." - Dr. Meera Shah, Nova IVF, Mountain View

The jury's out on these supplements often linked to fertility

There is a slew of other fertility-related supplements that are touted about on the internet, some of which are proven and *most are not*. Women often ask us about them, so we've included a brief overview of the existing research in order for you to make your own decision. Make sure to always check with your doctor before considering any of these supplements.

L-arginine

Current status: inconsistent evidence
Supplementation of this amino acid prior to ovarian stimulation is contentious. Some fertility specialists recommend it as a way to improve ovarian response, specifically for poor responders. ("Poor responders" are typically of advanced maternal age or have a low ovarian reserve.)[1031] Evidence for this recommendation comes from one study of 34 women in 1999, which suggested that supplementation of 16g/day of L-arginine could improve ovarian response prior to IVF treatments specifically for poor responders.[1032] However, a more recent double blind, randomized study by the same researchers found that women supplemented with the same amount had *lower* quality eggs retrieved, citing that it could be "detrimental to embryo quality."[1033] Subsequently, a study in 2010 found that women with more l-arginine in their bodies had fewer eggs retrieved during IVF and lower pregnancy rates (though the women were not taking l-arginine as a supplement).[1034]

Vitamin D

Current status: No cause-effect relationship established.

While getting healthy doses of vitamin D through sun exposure and food is undeniably good for you, recommendations on supplementation are still mixed. A large body of evidence now suggests it *does* have a beneficial impact on PCOS, endometriosis and IVF outcomes. However, studies suggest that vitamin D could exert positive effects on IVF outcomes through the womb, rather than through the quality of the eggs, so taking supplements of this vitamin might be more applicable for women trying to conceive, rather than egg freeze.[1035] [1036] [1037] If you don't get much time in the sun, or if you have trouble getting vitamin D through your diet, supplementation does offer a solution. But first, check to see if your prenatal vitamin includes it already.

DOCTOR PERSPECTIVE: "I check the vitamin D levels on all of my patients and prescribe a supplement as needed." - Dr. Diana Chavkin, HRC Fertility, Los Angeles

EXPERT INSIGHT: "In my experience, it can take up to three months for vitamin D levels to become sufficient. If a patient is taking a vitamin D supplement, I recommend she take her supplement along with a source of fat (i.e. yogurt, handful of almonds, cheese or avocado with toast). Vitamin D is a fat-soluble vitamin and the body absorbs fat-soluble vitamins more effectively if fat is on board. I usually recommend Vitamin D3 2000IU daily. However, if a patient is deficient, she may require a higher dosage. When choosing a supplement, I recommend cholecalciferol or vitamin D3 because these formats are more readily absorbed and effective compared to ergocalciferol or vitamin D2." - Elizabeth Stanway-Mayers, Clinical Dietitian, Stanford University Medical Center

Vitamin E

Current status: More evidence required.

Vitamin E has been shown to exhibit beneficial effects as an antioxidant within the ovaries, by protecting eggs from oxidative stress.[1038] This comes from a study in which certain levels of vitamin E in follicular fluid was associated with more mature eggs are retrieved. Similarly, with certain levels of vitamin E in blood, the results suggested, better quality embryos can be retrieved.[1039] In women over 35 years of age, supplementation with high doses of vitamin E was linked to better results in

IVF.[1040] [1041] However, as with vitamin D, it is thought the benefit could be primarily to the womb.[1042] Studies are still lacking.[1043]

Vitamin C

Current status: More evidence required.

Another antioxidant, vitamin C, is found in the ovaries so logic compels scientists to believe it plays a protective role against oxidative stress.[1044] But studies on the effect of vitamin C on fertility have mostly been either supplemented alongside other antioxidants, making it hard to isolate it's incremental effect, and/or they've been conducted on mice in which high doses not recommended for humans were administered. With that caveat in mind, a few studies have shown that vitamin C supplementation could counteract ovarian aging, resulting in more, higher quality eggs.[1045] [1046]

One study did find two months of vitamin C supplementation of 1000mg daily improved egg and embryo quality for women with endometriosis, though the study had only a small sample size.[1047] Another study found that non-smoking women who supplemented with 500 mg of vitamin C prior to IVF had a higher pregnancy rate than those that didn't.[1048] That said, your prenatal vitamin is likely to have some vitamin C so single supplementation is probably not needed.

Iron

Current status: More evidence required.

Multiple studies have shown that iron may be involved in ovulatory function and fertility.[1049] [1050] [1051] An observational study found a 40% lower risk of ovulatory infertility in women who took iron supplements.[1052] Also, findings from several studies suggest that women with celiac disease, which is usually linked with depletion of iron stores, as well as other micronutrients deficiencies, have impaired reproductive function.[1053]

Resveratrol

Current status: More evidence required.

This natural, highly-effective antioxidant mostly found in the peel and core of grapes, giving rise to "one glass of red wine for good health" mantra.[1054] Preliminary studies on animals and humans suggest that resveratrol could slow ovarian ageing and preserve egg quality for longer.[1055] [1056] But further tests in humans are required.

Catechins (+Quercetin / OPC)

Current status: More evidence required.

Catechins are antioxidants found in, for instance, green and matcha tea. They show a promising role in female fertility but the benefits are far from proven. More studies are needed.[1057]

Diosgenin

Current status: More evidence required.

Studies in mice suggest diosgenin, which is found in yams (tuber vegetables, similar to potatoes), could play a role in improved ovarian reserve by increasing the number of primary follicles and AMH levels.[1058] Of anecdotal interest, a 2011 study found that Central Africa has the highest rates of twin births in the world. A town in Nigeria, 142km north of Lagos, called Igbo-Orain, is commonly known as "the land of twins" because of the very high rate of twin pregnancies. While the researchers identified increased maternal age as the most important factor, the Yoruba people that live there believe that their high yam consumption is the cause. Indeed, the crop is hugely common across Central Africa. While there is no evidence that eating lots of yams increases the likelihood of twin births, it is thought their diosgenin content - a natural plant estrogen - could potentially stimulate multiple ovulation.[1059] At this time there are no randomized, controlled, large scale human studies.

Pycnogenol

Current status: No thorough testing.

This antioxidant is extracted from pine bark, and thus is not found naturally in the body. This patented product has not been extensively tested for safety or efficacy.[1060]

Maca

Current status: More evidence required.

Maca, also known as Peruvian ginseng, has a reputation for being an aphrodisiac. Animal studies suggest there might be some benefits to fertility. One study found that supplementing mice with yellow maca resulted in an increased litter size compared to those that weren't.[1061] But results from human studies are mixed and mostly involve improvements to sperm quality.[1062]

Chinese herbs

Current status: More evidence required.

Traditional Chinese medicine falls under the bracket known as "complementary and alternative medicines," or CAMs. A recent review of the body of literature found that studies have many shortcomings, such as small size, low quality, and lack of uniform standards in clinical trials. The kind of high-quality evidence required for clinical application has not been met, though it shows some promise.[1063]

Supplements to avoid

Some of the criticism leveled at supplements is that they can do more harm than good and, in the case of a few, that's a warning we should heed. It's not worth risking the outcome of your egg freezing procedure by taking supplements that have been scientifically shown to have potentially negative effects, or where the effects are unclear, even if hearsay says otherwise. Here are the ones doctors routinely advise giving a miss:

Royal Jelly

Current status: Testing in humans needed. May have adverse effects.

Royal jelly, a substance secreted by worker bees in order to provide food for the queen bee, is often touted as a "fertility superfood." It is packed with amino acids, lipids, sugars, vitamins, fatty acids, iron and calcium. In rats, it has been shown to improve follicle growth. However it also increases levels of steroid hormones[1064] and has an estrogenic effect.[1065] It's thought to help with fertility because of the mix of chemicals that act like hormones, but this can have an unpredictable effect and disrupt natural hormone balance.[1066] It also contains some of the same allergens found in bee venom and some life-threatening allergic reactions have been reported.[1067]

Chasteberry (chastetree, chastetree berry, Vitex, monk's pepper, lilac chastetree)

Current status: Avoid for egg freezing. May have adverse effects.

This supplement is often used to try to prevent miscarriages linked to low progesterone.[1068] A double-blind study conducted at Stanford found that chasteberry, green tea, vitamin E and vitamin B6, in combination, improved chances of conception.[1069] However, it is hard to separate out the individual benefits it confers, and as it could have an effect on hormonal balance, chasteberry is not recommended for use prior to or during ovarian stimulation.

St. John's Wort and other common drugstore herbal remedies

Current status: Avoid for egg freezing.

St John's Wort (a popular herbal mood enhancer) may have adverse effects on eggs.[1070] This was also true for Echinacea and ginkgo biloba.

OBLIGATORY DISCLAIMER: This list is not exhaustive and you should check with your doctor before taking any supplements, even those which are naturally derived.

HOW TO: Buy the best brands and bottles

A simple stroll down the supplements section of any drugstore or scroll online is so packed with options, it's enough to leave you in complete decision-making paralysis. Sometimes it's tempting just to give up trying to differentiate the brands and just buy *anything* to get it done. The thing is, the type, dosage, source and quality of the supplements you buy *really does matter*. Think of it this way, if you're going to spend the time and money to buy them in the first place, you might as well get the ones that could actually work. Without sufficient levels of the right ingredients, it's not worth taking them at all. Furthermore, some of the "bad actors" in the under-regulated supplements industry could be adding or altering the formulas in a way that might actually be harmful. So, with your safety, egg freezing outcome and bank balance in mind, we've put together a checklist of attributes to look for in a supplement.

Approach supplement brands with some skepticism

Despite the US supplements market being valued at $130 billion, they remain pretty controversial.

Supplements are not licensed or regulated like medicines, despite their ability to impact our health. That's because, unlike medications, supplements are classified as foods, not drugs. The regulatory guidelines for foods are much looser than those for medications. The Food & Drug Administration (FDA) is not required to regulate the ingredients or the efficacy of something sold as a supplement, nor does a supplement company need to show proof of a manufacturers' license as it would for medications.[1071] Basically, they are not controlled or monitored any more thoroughly than a Diet Coke. There is, therefore, a greater opportunity for unscrupulous supplement suppliers to sell bad or harmful products or products that are essentially useless, than if these products were monitored like drugs. With this in mind, it should come as no surprise that many public health experts are calling for the FDA to be given more teeth to police supplements. In the absence of this, later in this chapter we'll arm you with some key questions that can help you do your own detective work and find the best supplements:

Supplement quality control assessment criteria

When you pick up a supplement bottle (or click on the page link), there are a few criteria that can help you assess whether or not the contents of the bottle deliver on their claims, that they don't have other harmful or unnecessary substances, and that they offer the nutritional levels that you want.

1. Has it been validated by a credible third party?

Just because something is on a drugstore shelf does not mean it is what it says it is. One study tested the supplement myo-inositol and found concentrations to be 25% less than the labeling amount.[1072] Another study reviewed the contents of 44 herbal supplements sold in the US and found that 60% of them had ingredients not listed on the label, including fillers and cheaper substitutes.[1073] But there are certain precautions you can take to ensure that you're getting what you pay for.

First, look for a product that has been manufactured at a Good Manufacturing Practices (GMP) facility. A GMP-approved facility must comply with high standards, the same standards mandated by the US Food and Drug Administration for pharmaceutical manufacturers, which ensures that supplements are free from contamination and are accurately labeled. You can also look for trusted quality assurance companies such as NSF International, US Pharmacopeia, Underwriters Laboratory, or ConsumerLab seal. These verify that the product actually contains the ingredients that the label says it does, and that the product doesn't have any potentially harmful ingredients. Another online resource for cross-checking the quality of a supplement is Labdoor. This independent research lab takes popular supplements off the shelf and sends them to FDA registered labs for analysis at which point they are given a quality ranking score.

Also, be wary of supplements made outside the United States. Many aren't regulated, and some may have toxic ingredients.

The FDA is currently attempting to strengthen regulation by expanding its oversight.[1074] At least somewhat reassuringly, if a product is found to be unsafe after it hits the market, the FDA does have the power to restrict or ban its use.[1075] [1076] The takeaway here is that just because a supplement is on a shelf or doesn't require a prescription, that doesn't automatically make it safe or effective.

2. Is there enough of the desired ingredient?

All dietary supplements are required to have a "Supplement Facts" panel that lists the contents of each pill, which includes the amount of active ingredients per serving. This is the first place you want to look in order to make sure you're getting the amount of the ingredient desired (If you buy supplements online, make sure they show a photo of the Supplement Facts panel for you to review.) Keep in mind that these amounts apply to a single pill, so multiple servings might be necessary to get to the right amount.

Pay extra attention when buying prenatal vitamins in which multiple ingredients are combined into one pill. Many companies will lump a bunch of them together at the bottom of the label, usually under the title "proprietary blend" in a marketing effort to add to the appeal to shoppers. More often than not, the ingredients inside this section aren't supplied in significant dosages to deliver any real benefit. This practice so prevalent, the industry has made a term for it: "fairy dusting."[1077]

Supplement Facts

Serving Size

Amount Per Serving		% DV
Zinc	8mg	62%
Vitamin B12	2.6mcg	214%
Folic Acid	600mcg	100%
Selenium	60mcg	86%
Iodine	200mcg	69%
Ubiquinol	100mg	N/A
Melatonin	3mg	N/A
Omega-3	1400mg	N/A

Proprietary Blend: This is often where ingredients are listed that aren't supplied in sufficient amounts deliver any real benefit. There's even an industry term for this called, "fairy dusting."

Other Ingredients: This is often where ingredients such as binders, coatings, colorings, and flavorings are listed. The worst ones include titanium dioxide and magnesium stearate.

3. Are there any harmful, "other ingredients" listed?

The FDA requires supplement labels to list all inactive, "other ingredients," which can be found in small print at the bottom of the label.[1078] These ingredients include binders, coatings, colorings, and flavorings. Some are necessary to make a neat pill and others allow it to be easily swallowed, but there are some which are unnecessary and even unhealthy. Here are a couple of the contentious ones:

- **Magnesium stearate** - (also called octadecanoic acid or magnesium salt) is a chalk-like substance used as a "flow agent" to keep supplements from sticking to production machinery and to prevent powder from clumping inside capsules. Magnesium stearate has become hugely controversial, partly over claims that it may affect your body's ability to properly absorb the very nutrients you are trying to get from the supplement![1079] However, to date there is no human data related to magnesium stearate toxicity.[1080] Its safety was most recently reviewed at the 2015 meeting of the Joint FAO/WHO Expert Committee on Food Additives and the opinion was that magnesium stearate is not toxic.[1081] [1082] Still, if you prefer to use a brand that substitutes it for a natural lubricant, look for bottles that are labeled "no magnesium stearate" and "no stearic acid."

- **Titanium Dioxide** - Often used as a pigment in vitamins and supplements to make them white, titanium dioxide has been linked to a number of problems including DNA damage, chronic fatigue, and fibromyalgia.[1083] Furthermore, animal studies have shown that it may even be a human carcinogen.[1084] A recent review found that existing toxicity studies cannot completely exclude human health risks and more research is needed.[1085] Look for supplements that use natural ingredients, such as turmeric, for color instead.

4. Does it come from natural or synthetic sources?

As with nutrients from food, natural vitamin forms extracted directly from plant material are generally more useful to your body than synthetic vitamins. "Natural" vitamins tend to include the important transporters, co-factors, and enzymes that help your body metabolize the nutrients just as if you were getting them through food. On the other hand, synthetics are completely "isolated" in their production, which means that all of those added resources are lost.

The extent to which synthetic nutrients are absorbed and used in the body compared to their natural counterparts is unknown[1086] but preliminary studies on specific nutrients, such as vitamin E, show that natural versions are absorbed twice as efficiently as the synthetic version.[1087]

When to start and stop taking supplements

If you wish to supplement your diet, it is a good idea to start taking supplements at least three to four months prior to your estimated egg retrieval date, if your timescale allows. First, this means your eggs get the right support at the time they are undergoing the critical phase of chromosomal processing and explosive growth. Second, some of the supplements mentioned will take a few months to take effect. This is especially true for Coenzyme Q10. That said, if you don't have three to four months, there may be some benefits to be found in taking them for a shorter period of time. If you have a particular medical reason to freeze your eggs as quickly as possible, don't unnecessarily delay your procedure.

During the actual 8-14 days of hormonal stimulation, the small pool of evidence points to the key supplements above being generally safe, if not beneficial. However, make sure to check with your doctor as there are always exceptions and this might vary depending on your own medical history and circumstances.

Key takeaways for supplements

Despite the fact that you don't need a prescription for most supplements, taking pills of any kind is not something that should be done without proper thought. Follow dosage instructions and remember - it is possible to "overdose" on some vitamins and minerals and experience some unwanted side effects (for instance, "selenium poisoning").

CONSIDER SUPPLEMENTING YOUR DIET WITH THE FOLLOWING		
Vitamin	**Other names / notes**	**Dosage**
Folic Acid	The synthetic form of folate (also known as vitamin B9). Often included as part of a prenatal vitamin	600mcg
Vitamin B12	Other names are cyanocobalamin or methylcobalamin. Can take as part of a prenatal or B-complex.	2.6mcg
Zinc	Other names are zinc gluconate, zinc sulfate and zinc acetate. Can take as part of a prenatal.	8mg (12mg for vegetarians)
Selenium	Often included as part of a prenatal vitamin.	60mg
Iodine	Often included as part of a prenatal vitamin.	150mcg
Ubiquinol	Coenzyme Q10 and ubiquinone are not as absorbable. Take in the morning with food.	100mg
Omega 3s	Look for supplements with sufficient EPA & DHA. Algal oil for vegetarians. Take with foods containing fat.	1400mg
Melatonin	Take at the same time every evening.	3mg

A downloadable version of this supplement checklist is available at elanzawellness.com.

- For women with PCOS, talk to your doctor about supplementing with myo-inositol and alpha-lipoic acid.

- For women with diminished ovarian reserve, talk to your doctor about supplementing with DHEA.

- If possible, start taking supplements three to four months prior to your estimated egg retrieval procedure

- The type, dosage, source and quality of the supplements you buy really does matter. Get the best ones by asking the following questions: Has it been reviewed and approved by a credible 3rd party? Does it have the desired dosage listed on the "Supplement Facts" label? Was it manufactured in the US? Does it contain potentially harmful ingredients, such as magnesium stearate or titanium dioxide, listed in the "other ingredients" section of the label? Is it derived from natural or synthetic sources?

- Always check with your doctor for any adverse reactions or issues with your existing medications prior to intake.

Chapter 10: Avoiding Hazards for Egg Health

"Prevention is better than cure."

-Erasmus

Take a look around you right now. What are you touching? What did you wash your hair with this morning? What products did you put on your face and body? What cleaning products are sitting under your kitchen sink? Chances are, they all have one thing in common: synthetic chemicals. The sheer volume of them that we're exposed to on a daily basis is nothing short of staggering, because they are *literally everywhere*. Certainly not all of them are harmful, in fact, they're rather useful for all sorts of reasons; however, scientists have uncovered a few chemicals lurking in everyday products that could be toxic to your reproductive health, both in the short and the long term.[1088][1089][1090][1091][1092][1093]

In fact, many scientists now believe that the vast and growing use of noxious substances in the typical modern home and workplace could be partly to blame for the widespread decline in fertility for both women and men.[1094][1095][1096][1097][1098][1099][1100][1101][1102] The full extent of the damage they can cause is still being discovered.[1103]

Fortunately, simply by being aware of what chemicals to look for and where they can be found will help you reduce your exposure and the harmful effects they have on your fertility.

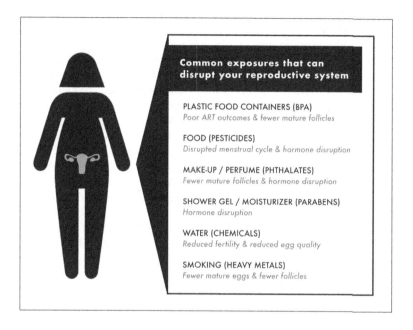

If some chemicals are so bad, why are they on the market?

This is the first question on most people's lips. Surely, if a chemical has made it into all kinds of products we touch and use every day of our lives, it must have gone through rigorous testing and government approvals, right? Well...not exactly.

Not all dangerous chemicals get banned

There are an estimated 85,000 man-made chemicals in the world, many of which you come into contact with every day.[1104] But only about one percent of these chemicals have actually been studied for safety. One percent! This happens even despite the fact that over 1,000 of them have known hormone-disrupting properties.[1105]

In the US, many of the chemicals and toxins in products do not get thoroughly studied or checked by regulatory agencies like the Environmental Protection Agency (EPA) until *after* they hit the market, if at all.[1106] Under existing US federal laws, chemical manufacturers are seldom required to provide the federal government with the necessary information to assess the safety of a chemical, even if it's new to the market.[1107]

Remember when lead paint and asbestos were once commonplace in homes across the globe?[1108] [1109]

And, as you might suspect, the chemicals that do get taken off the market tend to be those that create dramatic short term problems. But when it comes to chemicals and your reproductive system, the harmful impact might be longer term. If harm isn't seen immediately, it can be harder to find the source. This makes it a tough area to thoroughly study and has resulted in some conflicting results.[1110] It's also incredibly hard to separate out the effects of one single chemical except in short term lab conditions. The reality is, we encounter many chemicals, all at once, in concert. What this means is that the chemicals found in our homes, schools, workplaces, and communities have undergone only limited, if any, scrutiny in terms of their toxic effects on the reproductive system, especially over the medium to long term.[1111] [1112]

Even branding terms like "clean" and "natural" on labels are only loosely regulated and often don't translate to anything at all. This means that you have to do your homework by carefully reading through the lists of ingredients in order to find quality products that don't compromise your health. We will discuss this later - what to avoid and how to play toxin detective.

Household cleaning products are not required to list their ingredients

Unlike food, drugs and cosmetics, companies are not legally required to list out the ingredients on the labels of everyday household products unless they include "chemicals of known concern." Manufacturers lobby to keep it this way, arguing that revealing their ingredients will reveal their proprietary formulas to the competition. Whatever the reason, lack of transparency around the chemicals we are exposed to through our cleaning supplies makes it much harder to control our own health environment. One simple thing you can do is look out for an official consumer protection labeling system, if your country has one. In the US, this is the "Safer Choice Label" on household cleaning products. This stamp was created by the EPA as a way of indicating that the chemicals used have been deemed "safer."[1113]

Chemical safety tests are not conducted on women

Even when a chemical has been deemed safe, that doesn't necessarily mean it's been deemed safe for *you*, as a woman. There's a so-called "research gender gap" at play, whereby most chemical safety testing is conducted on a so-called *"Reference Man"* - that's to say, a 154 lb. (70kg)

Caucasian male, aged 25 to 30.[1114] Chances are, this doesn't accurately describe you. Or the majority of people, for that matter! That's some real white, male privilege with a dose of ageism thrown in for good measure. Why does it matter that this is the reference for chemicals testing tolerances? Because, the fact is, your body has a lower tolerance for chemicals than a man's. That's because your immune system and hormones, which can play a role in how chemicals are absorbed, are different. As with other women, you are also likely to be physically smaller and have thinner skin, both of which can lower the level of toxins you can be safely exposed to. Not only that, but chemicals can accumulate in body fat, which, yep, women also tend to have more of!

The campaigner Caroline Criado-Perez, who first uncovered and wrote about this issue, also points out that there is a systemic failure to adequately research female bodies, occupations and environments (for instance, nail salons and cleaning products) that may be affected by chemicals exposures on par with traditionally male-dominated ones (things such as mining and manufacturing).[1115] This means that there's a lack of data for exactly what could be causing the noticeable rise of diseases like breast cancer and - to our point - infertility. The takeaway here is to be aware that there aren't as many guardian angels watching over your chemical exposure as you might hope and assume.

So what can you do about it?

It starts right here. In this chapter you'll get to know which chemicals pose the biggest threat to your ovaries and maturing eggs. After doing a quick assessment of your makeup drawer, bathroom, kitchen, and aspects of your daily routine, you'll be able to identify the most toxic products and activities, which, over time, you can swap out for others that are less likely to cause harm.

Bisphenol-A (BPA)

BPA is most famously known as the "gender-bending" chemical due to its effects on male breast growth (or, as you might know them, "man boobs") [1116] and reduced penis size in newborn male infants.[1117] But more on the subject of you, BPA exposure is consistently linked to negative reproductive outcomes such as fewer eggs retrieved, fewer mature eggs and fewer fertilized eggs for women undergoing IVF.[1118][1119][1120][1121] In fact, 139 different research studies indicate that BPA disrupts the egg maturation process and reduces egg quality.[1122][1123]

Where is BPA found?

So, what actually *is* this three letter foe? BPA is a chemical used to bring transparency, colorability and flexibility to plastics, while also making them hard, watertight and shatterproof. BPA is also used to make epoxy resins, which are put on the inner lining of canned food containers to keep the metal from corroding and breaking.[1124] So, pretty useful, and you can see why it's everywhere. But there's an alarming cost to this level of reliance on BPA within the food and packaging industries - it can leach out of canned food linings and into food, or out of plastic food storage containers, especially when heated.[1125] That makes diet the main source of BPA exposure.[1126] BPA can enter your body through your stomach in food you've eaten, or merely through contact with your skin. It's hardly a shock, then, that data indicates that measurable levels of BPA are found in more than 90% of the US population.[1127]

What the science says about BPA

BPA is far from being a lone wolf terrorist - it's part of a wider cell of toxic substances known as endocrine disrupting chemicals (EDCs). The word "endocrine" is a fancy way of talking about hormones. EDCs disrupt your hormones by masquerading as one of them, which can enhance, dampen, or block the action of the actual hormones your body secretes naturally.[1128] [1129] This is problematic because your body can't tell the difference between the real and the fake, which throws off that very delicate hormonal balance that is required for your reproductive system to function properly.[1130] This hormonal disruption is no joke. Studies indicate that EDCs like BPA are linked to a host of female reproductive dysfunctions such as early puberty, infertility, abnormal menstrual cycles, premature ovarian failure/menopause, endometriosis, fibroids and adverse pregnancy outcomes.[1131] [1132] [1133] [1134] [1135] [1136] [1137] [1138] [1139] [1140] [1141] [1142]

In fact, The Endocrine Society believes it's no coincidence that declining sperm counts (up to 50% in the last half century[1143]), earlier puberty in girls worldwide, and genital malformations in people and animals coincide with the 500% rise in the amount of plastics (which BPA is often found in) produced since the 1970s -[1144] though that's nearly impossible to even try to prove.

BPA, in particular, mimics estrogen. In fact, BPA was originally studied as a potential source of synthetic estrogen before manufacturers started using it to make plastics(!)[1145] Wow.

It seems crazy that it wasn't banned long ago, as BPA's influence on fertility was actually first uncovered as long as twenty years ago. Albeit on mice. The link was actually discovered inadvertently. Researchers were studying the reproductive systems of female mice to gather data on other fertility issues, when they discovered female mice were developing chromosomally abnormal eggs among a host of other unexpected fertility issues.[1146] They eventually isolated the source to BPA leaching out of plastic mouse cages, which the mice had damaged through chewing. They repeated the experiment, and found that in the female mice, even short-term, low-dose exposure during the final stages of egg growth was sufficient to show detectable effects.

But, why isn't it banned?

Despite some powerful evidence, the US Food and Drug Administration (FDA) maintains that the amount of BPA leaching from food packaging will not harm people.[1147] But this begs the question of why BPA has been banned in the manufacturing of baby bottles and sippy cups in many countries around the world.[1148] The FDA does say that there is "some concern about the potential effects of BPA on the brain, behavior and prostate glands of fetuses, infants and children." As of 2019, BPA has faced some restrictions in the EU[1149] and Canada,[1150] but in the US, the subject is a matter of contentious debate. There is of course massive political pressure from the polycarbonate, metal packaging and food industries, which profit from the eight billion pounds of BPA produced annually.[1151 1152 1153]

One reason the FDA has not outright banned BPA is because of the findings from a large three-agency study called "CLARITY-BPA." The study authors concluded that BPA exposure up to 50 micrograms per day is safe. However, biologists from a slew of American universities completely disagree, saying that even low-dose BPA exposure causes health issues, with the greatest number of problems observed at doses 20,000 micrograms *lower* than the dose the FDA currently considers "safe" for humans.[1154] It's worth pointing out that of the studies funded by the chemical industry, 100% concluded that BPA causes no significant effects.[1155] In contrast, 92% of the studies not funded by industry found did find significant negative effects of BPA exposure.

While there is still room for debate on the level at which BPA becomes toxic, we do know is that even small changes to our hormones can have large biological effects. This fact alone has lead scientists to think that BPA exposures, even at low doses, can disrupt the body's delicate endocrine system and lead to many adverse effects.[1156 1157] This feels particularly significant when you consider that the egg and its "meiotic spindle" (the part involved in critical DNA processes) are sensitive to hormone changes.

How to avoid BPA

While it's almost impossible to completely eliminate BPA from your environment, you can make more conscious choices about the foods you eat, beverages you drink and things you touch. The good news is that by making these changes, your body will be able to start eliminating BPA from your system within a matter of days.[1158]

- **Avoid using plastic items in the kitchen, even if it says "BPA-free"** - In light of the concern around BPA, manufacturers have replaced it with similar chemicals called bisphenol-S (BPS) and bisphenol-F (BPF) that can be equally as damaging, even in small concentrations.[1159 1160]

- **Reduce consumption of foods packaged and stored in plastic** - Avoid plastic items labeled with the recycling numbers 3 and 7 or the letters "PC," which likely contain BPA, BPS or BPF.

- **Throw out old and scratched plastic items** – BPA is more likely to leach into food and beverages through tiny cracks and crevices in plastics.

- **Replace plastic Tupperware with glass** - BPA leaches into food over time so food stored in plastic is likely to soak up more of this toxin.

- **Don't heat up plastic** - Don't put plastic containers in the microwave or wash them at very high temperatures. BPA is more likely to leach into your food.

- **Don't consume foods from cans** - BPA is often found in the lining of cans.[1161] Not all cans are lined with it, but it's impossible for you to tell whether or not it does from the label. Play it safe by buying fresh foods or buying those packaged in glass or paper instead. For drinking on the go, look for stainless steel bottles that do not have a liner. Some metal water bottles lined with an epoxy-based enamel coating could leach BPA. If you do eat fruit or vegetables from a can, research indicates that rinsing them before eating may reduce the amount of BPA you ingest.[1162]

- **Say "no" to printed receipts** - Thermal paper is often coated with BPA, so ask for your receipt to be emailed or forego it altogether, where possible. If you handle receipts as part of your job, wash your hands thoroughly before eating, or consider wearing gloves.[1163 1164]

- **Stay hydrated** - Drinking at least half your body weight in ounces of clean, purified or filtered water daily will help flush out environmental hazards (as well as improving your circulation, which helps hormones travel to where they're needed throughout the body). For example, if you weigh 120 pounds, you should drink 60 ounces of water, or about 1.8 quarts.[1165] Even being slightly dehydrated can sabotage your body by affecting hormone balance, the concentration of toxins in your bloodstream and nutrient absorption. Long-term disturbances due to lack of hydration in the tissue can result in oxidative stress and in extreme cases lead to DNA damage and permanent cellular dysfunction.[1166]

Phthalates

You'll never see this hard to pronounce word, phthalates (*"fthal-eights"*) on a label. That's because it's not one specific chemical, but rather, a catch-all term that encompasses a vast group of synthetic chemicals. Most of these, surprise-surprise, have never even been studied for safety. Several of those that have been examined indicate negative repercussions for your delicate eggs.

Where are phthalates found?

Phthalates enjoy widespread global production in excess of 18 billion pounds per year.[1167] They are mostly used as plasticizers, added to plastic resins in effort to increase flexibility. They are also used as solvents, adhesives, defoaming agents, and lubricants in a vast array of products, making them particularly hard to eliminate.[1168 1169 1170] Just today, you've probably been exposed phthalates purely by eating, drinking, breathing, and wearing any type of personal care product or cosmetic.

Phthalates are similar to BPA in the sense that they can leach from their intended host into your food, as well as the atmosphere (some bind to dust particles), soil and groundwater.[1171 1172 1173]

75–100% of the population is exposed to phthalates on a daily basis.[1174 1175 1176] But women of reproductive age tend to have the highest exposure levels to a phthalate known as "MBP" compared to any other age/sex group, most likely due to its usage in cosmetics and personal care products.[1177] Despite its ubiquity within female-oriented products, there is almost no understanding of the degree to which MBP's are damaging to women. This is particularly concerning to women that are frequently exposed to phthalates at their jobs, for instance in nail salons or house cleaning. And the bulk of the research, where it exists, only looks at absorption through the skin, rather than through other exposures such as, as in the nail salon example, inhaling filing dust or fumes from nail polish remover.[1178]

What the science says about phthalates

Due to their ubiquity in the environment, phthalates are of significant concern to scientists and yet there is still very little known about the potential short and long-term repercussions on women's fertility, not to mention overall health.[1179] Initial studies conducted on mice link phthalates' toxic effects to premature ovarian failure, anovulation, infertility, and decreased sex hormone production.[1180 1181 1182 1183]

The reason this happens - and most relevant to the results of your egg freezing outcome - is that phthalates can target your eggs at a particular stage of growth, at which point they can prevent your eggs from maturing and reduce the total number of follicles in your ovaries. This is possible because of a dual attack on your eggs, first disrupting your hormones - putting it in the endocrine disruptor (EDC) category - and then by increasing the level of oxidative stress on your ovaries.[1184 1185 1186 1187] As such, exposure to these chemicals could theoretically inhibit your growing eggs, reducing the quantity retrieved from your egg freezing procedure.[1188] And if exposure limits the growth of your eggs, they would not be able to reach maturity in time to be deemed of a quality worth freezing.[1189]

How to avoid phthalates

Full avoidance of phthalates may be impossible without institutional changes; however, there are day-to-day modifications you can make that will help reduce your exposure and reduce the existing build-up in your body.

- **Avoid products with fragrance or perfume**[1190] - Look for labels that say "phthalate-free" or "no synthetic fragrance" instead. Check out resources like the Environmental Working Group to see which ones pass the test.

- **Ditch fast food** - Opt for organic fruits and vegetables that aren't packaged in plastic.

- **Swap out plastic containers for glass or stainless steel -** Switch to glass and stainless containers and water bottles (also important for BPA). In particular, check the code on your plastic bottles—3 and 7 may have phthalates.

- **Only use "phthalate-free" sex toys from reputable manufacturers**[1191] - The sex toy industry goes largely unregulated, so if you use sex toys it pays to buy them from well-regarded companies. The membranes in intimate areas are very porous and can absorb chemicals more readily than the rest of your body.

Parabens

This is one you've probably heard of, thanks to widespread discussion of the effects of human exposure to parabens. But despite its reputation, the research on this chemical is less conclusive than for BPA or phthalates. Some of the extensive tests in animals that showed negative effects have not shown the same results in humans, which has led to some controversy within the scientific community as to what the measurable impact is on humans.[1192] [1193] [1194] What scientists do agree on is that parabens are considered endocrine disruptors due to their ability to mimic the estrogen hormone.

Where are they found?

Parabens are preservatives that are most commonly found in cosmetics and body care products in order to prevent the growth of mold and other harmful bacteria. They are also used as preservatives in food and beverages, as well as some medications in order to give them a longer shelf life.[1195] [1196] One study found parabens in nearly all urine samples from American adults, regardless of ethnic, socioeconomic or geographic backgrounds.[1197]

Parabens can enter the human body through the skin and by ingestion. Your average paraben exposure per day is estimated to be 76 mg.[1198] [1199] [1200] While FDA limits the levels of parabens allowed in foods and beverages, it does not regulate these chemicals in cosmetics and body care products.[1201] But unlike cleaning products, cosmetics and personal care items are required to list the ingredients on the label, which makes it a little easier to avoid them in the first place.

What the science says about parabens

Results from studies haven't painted a particularly clear picture as to the potential negative effects. One study, for example, found no connection between paraben level in urine samples and IVF outcomes,[1202] whereas another similar study did find a link between elevated paraben levels and poor embryo quality.[1203]

Scientists have even noted that the ovaries of young rats who were exposed to high doses of paraben exposure looked more like the ovaries of those who had already gone through menopause![1204] And in women, one study found that at least one paraben (propylparaben) may be linked to diminished ovarian reserve.[1205]

While there is still debate about the threshold of exposure that makes it hazardous to humans, parabens operate the same way as BPA, mimicking and blocking estrogen in your body. The results of this have been shown to disrupt early egg maturation by diminishing the amount of follicles (immature eggs) in your ovaries.[1206]

How to avoid parabens

Thanks to the growing body of data warning against the negative effects of parabens, many natural skincare, makeup and hair-care brands have altered their formulations to be "paraben free." But there are still many lurking out there.

Avoid personal care products with chemicals ending in "-paraben." - Cosmetics sold in stores or online must have a list of ingredients, each listed by its common or usual name. In most cases, you can be your own detective by looking for ingredients with -paraben at the end. Here are a few of the big ones.

- Methylparaben (alternative names are 4-hydroxy methyl ester benzoic acid and methyl 4-hydroxybenzoate)

- Ethylparaben

- Propylparaben

- Butylparaben

- Isobutylparaben

- Benzylparaben is less common

If you want to check for parabens in the products you already use (as often the ingredient list is only shown on the original packaging), check out the app "Think Dirty," or look for your cosmetics on the Skin Deep product database.

Be selective about sunscreen - One such product we can't (or shouldn't!) live without is sunscreen. It's good to get a little sunshine sometimes, as the best source of vitamin D. However, try to use sunscreens with natural, "mineral" formulations where zinc oxide is the active ingredient. They should be oil-free, non-comedogenic and should not have any oxybenzone, parabens, or other endocrine disruptors. The Environmental Working Group has a list of sunscreens that it approves.

Pesticides

Pesticides cover a range of chemical agents contained within products that kill everything from insects, fungus and weeds to rodents and other crop pests. Some studies have shown that the many chemicals found in pesticides can reduce your fertility in a few ways,[1207] both by disrupting your hormones and by damaging the structure of your cells.[1208]

What the science says about pesticides

Because pesticides cover a vast array of compounds and chemical combinations, it's hard to know which ones are the most damaging. Broadly, pesticides have been linked to a number of negative impacts on human health and wellbeing, evidenced most clearly by the higher rates of physical and mental health problems (such as Parkinson's disease and depression/suicide in agricultural workers who are the most exposed to pesticides).[1209] [1210] [1211]

When it comes to fertility specifically, the data is limited for ethical reasons (we can't say we're in support of running a study that deliberately exposes women to pesticides). However, the data we do have does not look great. It's linked to a variety of reproductive issues and pregnancy outcomes such as ovarian disorders, miscarriage, stillbirth, premature birth, low birth weight, developmental abnormalities.[1212] [1213]

Scientists theorize that pesticides have the power to disrupt the hormonal function of the female reproductive system, which can cause adverse effects on the entire ovary. And, the disruption is thought to take place at multiple stages of follicle (egg) growth.[1214] If this is the case, it explains why test subjects exposed to pesticides exhibit a high incidence of cystic ovaries, inhibited follicle growth and decreased mature follicle count.[1215 1216 1217 1218 1219 1220 1221 1222 1223] In simple terms, this means that exposure to pesticides could reduce the number of mature eggs retrieved from your stimulation cycle. Exactly which pesticides, and at what levels, could have the most detrimental effect is still up for debate, but, logically, anything that's capable of shutting down the nervous system of an insect is something we want to minimize eating! If you work in an industry where you are exposed to pesticides (agriculture, landscape gardening) or you live in an agricultural area, avoiding further exposure through your food might be a particular concern for you.

Avoiding pesticides found in food

Fortunately, the US Environmental Protection Agency (EPA) and other agencies regulate pesticide residues in our food. Play it safe by making a few simple changes to avoid unnecessary exposure.

- **Eat a variety of fruits and vegetables** to minimize the potential of increased exposure to a single pesticide. However, some are considered more "dirty" than others. If financial or other restrictions limit your access to organic foods, remember to look to the "Clean 15" list (found in the "Eating for Egg Health chapter) to identify the produce with the lowest levels of pesticide exposure. Basically, don't avoid eating fruit or vegetables, just finesse your choices as best as possible.

- **Buy organic**, if possible.[1224]

- **Thoroughly wash or clean all produce,** even those labeled as "organic" and particularly if the item needs to be peeled. Pesticide residues on food decline over time as the food moves through various stages from the farm to your fridge, but they do still remain on some foods.[1225] Wash your produce under running water rather than soaking or dunking it. Scrub firm fruits and vegetables such as melons and root vegetables. Discard the outer layer of leafy vegetables such as lettuce or cabbage.

- **Trim fat and skin from meat, poultry, and fish** to minimize pesticide residue that may accumulate in the fat.

Avoiding pesticides found in drinking water

Some drinking water is a source of potentially damaging contaminants. When the US Geological Survey (USGS) conducted tests on water, including one study in nine states across the country, it found 85 man-made chemicals including traces of things like antibiotics, anticonvulsants, mood stabilizers and oral contraceptives.[1226 1227 1228] The

USGS claimed these were in such small amounts that they didn't pose health risks, however, researchers have found that even very diluted concentrations of drug residues can impair human cell function. While there are regulations around drinking water in the United States, some scientists believe that regulatory guidelines may sometimes fall short. This is partly due to a lack of sufficient data regarding the health hazards of chronic low dose exposure to contaminants, as well as the fact that new substances (pesticides, medications etc.) are regularly introduced that have not yet been properly studied. Each state in the US has its separate individual standards, which allows a significant variation in those standards.[1229] The EPA also regulates and monitors several drinking water contaminants, but many pesticides are not considered part of that list.[1230] Tap water suppliers in the US are required to publish their water quality tests every year, so you can look up your US city's report on the Environmental Working Group (EWC) National Tap Water Database.

- **Get a water filter** - It's not easy to remove birth control and other drugs from tap water. But the best suggested devices are a combination of charcoal and reverse-osmosis filters. Installing this just for drinking water is sufficient, as shower water is not generally ingested.

- **Make sure you change your water filters on time** - Old filters can harbor bacteria and let contaminants through.

- **Avoid bottled water** - Bottled water companies are not required to publish quality tests. You can read the bottle label and still not know whether the water is pure or just processed tap water. The EWG found 38 contaminants in 10 popular bottled water brands.[1231] If you're going to buy it, try to buy it in glass bottles.

Avoiding pesticides in the air[1232]

We're not saying live in a bubble, or walk around in a mask 24/7, but the very air we breathe is up for discussion. The toxicity of pesticides in the air is driven first by how toxic the pesticide is, then by how much of it is in the air and how much you breathe in or are exposed to. Research indicates low levels of pesticides are present in the air of many homes. This may be caused by using pesticides indoors and/or by contaminated dust, dirt and air entering the home from outside.

- **Avoid the use of all pesticides in your home(e.g. weed sprays, bug sprays, rodent killers, etc.)** - Antimicrobials and disinfectants are pesticides too. Use them only when needed and as directed. If you must use them, mix and dilute pesticides outside the home, even when treating indoors. Use chemical free cleaning solutions or make your own![1233] Take a look at our website for some more practical advice here.

- **Ventilate your home** - Good ventilation can reduce the concentration of pesticides.

- **Stay indoors if industrial pesticides are being deployed** - If you are in an agricultural area where pesticides are often used, monitor when they are being deployed and try to leave the area. Additionally, keep an eye out for very hot or windy days when they can be spread more easily.

- **Consider purchasing an air purifier** - While you're never going to be able to avoid certain airborne toxic exposures, things like traffic fumes, at least when and where you sleep you can breathe easy. For 8 hours a day, you can rest assured that you are inhaling clean air, especially if you live near fields that have recently been sprayed.

Heavy Metals

Heavy metals include metals such as lead, mercury, boron, aluminum, cadmium, arsenic, antimony, cobalt, and lithium. Although these elements are found in nature, the Occupational Safety & Health Administration warns that they can be harmful to your health, especially over a long period of time or in high doses.[1234] Some of these metals, such as zinc, copper, and iron, are good for you in small amounts, but overexposure can have a toxic effect on your ovaries caused by hormonal disruption.[1235] [1236]

We are exposed to a variety of heavy metals via everything from cigarettes and dietary supplements to contaminated food, air, and water.[1237] For example, cadmium is a heavy metal found abundantly within cigarette tobacco,[1238] which accumulates in the ovaries of habitual smokers over time.[1239] You can also be exposed to heavy metals through air pollution. Some estimates indicate that in the US, more than 100 to 200,000 tons of lead per year is released from vehicle exhausts.[1240]

EXPERT INSIGHT: "I recently discovered that a few of my 'healthy' food supplements, like organic, raw cacao were reported for containing heavy metals. If you want to take the extra step, you can reach out to companies and request their heavy metal reports. If they haven't conducted these types of inspections on their supplements, they probably aren't a trustworthy brand. 'Organic' unfortunately does not mean free of heavy metals." - Kaitlyn Noble, Pre and Post-natal Health Coach, Los Angeles

Why are they bad?

While research is limited, studies have confirmed that women with high levels of heavy metals such as lead and mercury tend to have significantly fewer of mature eggs retrieved in IVF.[1241] [1242] [1243] Research also indicates that cadmium,[1244] boron,[1245] and sodium arsenite[1246] can alter our reproductive hormones, of which the consequences on fertility are still being discovered.

A 2017 review found that studies in both animals and humans show air pollution causes defects in egg maturation and leads to a drop in reproductive capacity.[1247] It showed that particulate matter from, for example, diesel exhaust, can cause hormone disruption,[1248] [1249] [1250] [1251] that air pollution can generate oxidative stress[1252] [1253] [1254] and cause alterations in DNA, leading to mutations,[1255] [1256] [1257] [1258] [1259] which is why there are considerable concerns around fertility.

Emerging evidence suggests that babies developing in the womb may be particularly sensitive to maternal exposure to air pollutants.[1260] [1261] It's not too much of a stretch, given the other available evidence, to see that this could also apply to your developing eggs. While it can be difficult to eliminate these EDCs from our lives completely, awareness of the ways we come into contact with them can help us find ways to limit our exposure.

How to limit your exposure to heavy metals

- **Stop smoking and avoid secondhand smoke** - You can also be exposed to toxic metals in cigarette smoke.[1262] Smoking or being around others who smoke increases cadmium levels in your body.

- Wear personal protective equipment if you work in a place where heavy metals are used (e.g. batteries, metal coatings, and plastics) - Wear specialized protective equipment when necessary and always remove your work clothes and shower before returning home.

- **Stay indoors when pollution is highest, where possible** - Environmental protection agencies in most countries advise people to stay indoors as part of guidance to reduce exposure on high air pollution days.[1263] In the US, the EPA's *Air Quality Index* (AQI) includes "good, moderate, unhealthy for sensitive individuals, unhealthy, very unhealthy, and hazardous" bands, which you can check on their website.[1264]

- **Know that your exposure may be highest on sunny days** - Ambient air pollution levels vary by season, weather, events and time of day. One of the big factors is actually sunshine. That's because ultraviolet light from the sun activates the reactions that form ozone, a molecule harmful to air quality. That means there are usually higher concentrations of ozone in late morning to early evening.[1265] Basically, pollution can be higher on sunny days - exactly when everyone wants to be outside!

- **Breathe through your nose while sitting in traffic** - Your nose is a more effective natural air filter than your mouth, which means water-soluble gases and vapors are less likely to reach your lungs.[1266]

- **Avoid exercising outside on heavy smog days** - if you live in a place that has lots of smog, avoid extended outdoor activities when the rates are higher.[1267] Physical exertion will increase your breathing and opportunity to inhale harmful heavy metals.[1268]

- **Avoid exercising outside alongside heavy roadways** - You can avoid inhaling air pollutants by running, cycling, walking, etc. in less congested areas such as parks. Pollution concentrations fall rapidly starting about a third of a mile away from the traffic.[1269] If you do need to get active around traffic, for example, if you cycle to work, then you might consider one of the increasingly common respirators "face masks!" Their ability to remove contaminants does vary depending on fit, brand and type of filter, though, so make sure to buy from a reputable source.[1270]

- **Once again, consider a portable or central air purifying system** - These devices have been shown to reduce concentrations of indoor air pollutants, of either outdoor or indoor origin.[1271]

Medications and drugs

If you read the warning label on almost every over-the-counter medication, it will say something like, "If you're pregnant or breastfeeding, talk to your doctor." This message is partially for legal reasons, but it's also because scientists don't know for sure what the impact of every medication will be on fertility. There are a handful of studies that provide us with some insight as to which drugs might cause harm to your eggs, but considering the difficulties and ethics around measuring their impact, it's best to avoid taking a medication unless necessary or it is prescribed by a doctor.

Of course, if you are currently taking a medication, particularly a prescription drug, don't stop taking it without talking to your doctor first. It can be dangerous to discontinue some medications suddenly, and it may be better for you to continue taking it.

Anti-inflammatories (ibuprofen, paracetamol, acetaminophen)

Preliminary research shows that anti-inflammatories are capable of disrupting ovulation. This happens because ovulation involves a naturally inflammatory process in which the follicle in the ovary breaks open and releases an egg. The problem is that this "good" inflammation required for reproduction can be suppressed by the use of anti-inflammatory drugs, particularly prescription versions such as Indomethacin. That's why anti-inflammatory use can be a problem for women trying to get pregnant. Of course, for egg freezing you actually don't *want* to ovulate because your eggs will be retrieved and collected before this happens, so the thinking is that anti-inflammatories should not pose a problem, at least for most of the cycle. Speak to your doctor if you regularly take these medications, however.

DOCTOR PERSPECTIVE: "I usually tell my patients to stay away from these anti-inflammatory medications around the time of trigger shot and retrieval." - Dr. Diana Chavkin, HRC Fertility, Los Angeles

Skin drugs like Accutane

DOCTOR PERSPECTIVE: "[Ro]accutane is a vitamin A preparation used to treat severe acne. We suggest people do not use it for at least two months before trying for children. I would recommend holding off this treatment for this period of time before egg freezing, too, although there is no specific evidence in the literature against using it whilst undergoing ovarian stimulation. This also goes for the use of certain antibiotics and tablet therapy for conditions such as eczema and psoriasis. That's because certain medications take two to four months to come out of your system, including drugs like methotrexate, azathioprine and tetracyclines. So please seek advice from your dermatologist." Dr. Angela Tewari, Consultant Dermatologist, King's College Hospital, London

Psychiatric medications (e.g. antidepressants and antipsychotics)

Preliminary research indicates that these drugs can interfere with the hormonal regulation of ovulation and may also elevate the levels of hormones associated with ovulation, such as prolactin. One study showed that women who were taking SSRIs (selective serotonin reuptake inhibitors) took significantly longer to conceive.[1272] On the other hand, it is difficult to determine if this was due to the medication or due to other factors that could have played a role, such as underlying depression. Research is limited and, again, mostly involving ovulation itself. Always raise psychiatric conditions and medications with your doctor before starting ovarian stimulation hormones, so they can plan and balance the best course of action to keep you safe and healthy.

DOCTOR PERSPECTIVE: "It's important to weigh the risks and benefits of stopping psychiatric medications, so it is imperative to have this discussion with your doctor. In many cases, especially when medications are important for normal daily function and maintaining quality of life, they do not need to be stopped." - Dr. Meera Shah, Nova IVF, Mountain View

Steroids

It's thought that medications such as cortisone and prednisone, which are used to treat conditions including asthma and lupus, can prevent your pituitary gland from releasing enough follicle-stimulating hormone (FSH) and luteinizing hormone (LH) for normal ovulation, if taken in high doses. Research is limited, however, and points to an effect on ovulation itself rather than egg quality. Always talk to your primary care doctor with any concerns about your medication.

Opiates / opioids

In light of the "opioid crisis" in the US, there is a growing amount of research focused on the repercussions of opioids, both clinically and recreationally. Opioids operate as an endocrine disruptor by affecting the production of sex hormones. That is, when opioids are chronically present, the body has less ability to produce sufficient levels of crucial egg-quality hormones such as estrogen. Just a few of the issues linked to opioid use include loss of libido, menstrual irregularities and infertility.[1273] Discuss the options with your doctor who can suggest safe strategies for eliminating them, or for replacing them with over-the-counter painkillers.

Marijuana

The research on the impact of marijuana usage on egg quality and fertility is limited and inconclusive. Logically speaking, many of the harmful carcinogens found in cigarettes are also found in marijuana, which leads to the assumption that they are bad. Although a study back in the 1990's found women who smoked marijuana had an elevated risk of infertility due to lack of ovulation, as it appeared to interfere with hormone regulation,[1274] a recent analysis by the National Survey of Family Growth (NSFG) found no link.[1275] And another study showed that women who used marijuana at least once over a four year time frame had the same probability of getting pregnant as those who didn't.[1276] The ASRM take on it is that this study lays a good foundation for further investigation, but it does not constitute enough evidence to provide reassurance in and of itself. Still, the American College of Obstetricians and Gynecologists (ACOG) says marijuana use may have a harmful effect on reproduction in general terms[1277] and may be as harmful as tobacco. In short, limited research shows divided opinions on smoking marijuana.

Recreational drugs

Any doctor would advise you to eliminate the use of recreational drugs prior to your egg freezing procedure. Most human studies have looked at the effects on pregnancy and babies' development rather than on egg quality. However, a study conducted on mice showed that exposure to cocaine decreased egg quality.[1278] Women have more long-term physical effects from drugs (and alcohol) than men, thanks to differences in physiology, weight and hormone levels, and drug use may cause changes to the menstrual cycle.[1279] There are also suggestions that other lifestyle factors that impact fertility go hand in hand with drug use, such as low body weight and drinking more alcohol.

Pregnant women get high a lot more than you might think
In one survey, nearly five percent of the women admitted illicit drug use within the past 30 days,[1280] and in a drug screening of pregnant women in New Orleans, 19% of pregnant women tested positive for at least one illegal substance.[1281]

Other substances (Botox, fillers, hair dye)

There are some other popular beauty and cosmetic substances you might come into intimate contact with that would cause you concern if you were pregnant, so, should you be concerned about them before egg freezing?

DOCTOR PERSPECTIVE: "Botox and fillers are safe before egg freezing, as is hair dye. I tell women to avoid dyeing their hair during pregnancy, however." - Dr. Aimee Eyvazzadeh, Private Practice Physician, San Ramon

Key takeaways:

- Endocrine disrupting chemicals (EDCs) have the ability to disrupt your reproductive hormones and to damage your maturing eggs.

- In the US, many chemicals found in everyday products are not strongly regulated, which is why you need to be extra diligent about choosing products and taking actions that will reduce your chances of exposure.

- Hazardous chemicals to your fertility can be found in your cleaning products, kitchen tools and beauty products.

- Some of the most well-known chemicals to cause reproductive damage are:

- **BPA** - found in plastics, canned food containers, feminine hygiene products

- **Phthalates** - found in plastics, medication coatings, cosmetics with fragrance

- **Parabens** - found in cosmetics, toothpaste, processed food, face and hair care products

- **Pesticides** - found in drinking water, "dirty" foods, air supply near agricultural areas

- **Heavy metals** - Found in cigarettes, pollution, high mercury fish, household dust

- Make sure to review your entire medication list with your fertility doctor in case anything may interfere with the fertility drugs and your hormones and impact the success of your cycle.

- Avoid recreational drug use because the harmful effects are not fully understood.

CHECKLIST: AVOIDING HAZARDS FOR EGG HEALTH

Kitchen

- [ ] Ditch plastic items in the kitchen, even if it says "BPA-free" Check for the recycling numbers 3 and 7 or the letters "PC," as they likely contain BPA, BPA or BPF. Replace plastics with stainless steel or glass, especially if the plastic is old and scratched
- [ ] Don't heat up plastics in the microwave
- [ ] Avoid eating foods from cans If you do, wash them before eating
- [ ] Buy organic fruits and vegetables, if you can afford it
- [ ] Thoroughly wash all produce, especially those considered "dirty," even if they are organic
- [ ] Eat a variety of fruits and vegetables
- [ ] Trim fat and skin from meat, poultry, and fish
- [ ] Avoid eating fish known for their high levels of mercury, such as tuna
- [ ] Get a home water filter
- [ ] Avoid bottled water
- [ ] Look for cleaning products with the "Safer Choice Label"

Bathroom and makeup drawer

- [ ] Avoid products with fragrance or perfume
- [ ] Avoid personal care products with chemicals ending in "-paraben"
- [ ] Use sunscreens with natural, "mineral" formulations where zinc oxide is the active ingredient They should be oil-free, non-comedogenic and should not have any oxybenzone, parabens, or other endocrine disruptors

Rest of your home

- [ ] Avoid the use of all pesticides (e.g. weed sprays, bug sprays, rodent killers, etc.)
- [ ] Ventilate your home
- [ ] Stay indoors if industrial pesticides are being deployed
- [ ] Consider getting a portable or central air cleaning system

Out and about

- [ ] Say no to paper receipts
- [ ] Stay indoors when pollution is highest, where possible, especially on sunny days
- [ ] Breathe through your nose while sitting in traffic
- [ ] Avoid exercising outside on heavy smog days
- [ ] Avoid exercising outside alongside heavy roadways

A downloadable version of this checklist is available at
ELANZAwellness.com.

Chapter 11: Eggxercise

"The only way to make sense out of change is to plunge into it, move with it, and join the dance."

- Alan Watts

There's no such thing as a one-size-fits-all "prescription" for the right amount of exercise for egg health. That's because everyone's fitness baseline, lifestyle and physiological makeup are different. Striking the right balance between *how* you move, *how much* you move and *how many calories* you consume can support the functions needed to make healthy eggs. The crux of it is that too much or too little exercise could have a negative influence on your egg health.[1282]

In this chapter, you'll discover where you sit in the fertility "eggxercise" spectrum and how to adapt your levels and types of activity for each phase of the egg freezing journey.

Moderate exercise is the best for fertility

No matter what your current fitness level, moderate exercise is thought to benefit your hormone profile and reproductive function.[1283] The magic word here is *moderation*. We should mention that there isn't much research on the direct impact of moderate exercise on the outcomes of fertility treatments such as egg freezing. That said, many of the reproductive benefits associated with moderate exercise are linked to all kinds of factors that indirectly influence your fertility:

- **Improves blood flow to your reproductive organs** - During the ovarian stimulation phase, blood flow is one of the things your doctor will assess when scanning your ovaries. That's because good, oxygen-rich blood flow is vital for the growth process of the follicles that contain your maturing eggs.[1284] Good circulation is thought to have a positive effect on egg quality and success rates in ovarian stimulation. Experimental data has linked the number of eggs retrieved and the quality of eggs retrieved to ovaries with good blood flow.[1285] [1286] [1287] [1288]

- **Reduces oxidative stress**[1289] - Intense exercise generates a lot of free radicals, more than your body's antioxidant levels can balance out. But when you exercise in moderation, your body's antioxidant levels are able to rise enough to neutralize the damaging effects of free radicals and to protect against future attacks, particularly within the ovaries.[1290] [1291] [1292] [1293] [1294] [1295]

- **Helps maintain a healthy level of body fat** - As you might remember, women who are on the heavier side have a pregnancy rate that is 30%-75% below that of women who are not.[1296] [1297] [1298]

- **Helps manage blood sugar levels** - High blood sugar levels can significantly decrease both the quantity and quality of eggs retrieved in your egg freezing cycle.[1299] But research shows that moderate exercise can help improve insulin sensitivity and glycemic control.[1300] [1301] If you fall into the obese category, even a modest session of exercise is shown to improve insulin sensitivity.[1302]

- **Helps manage stress hormones** - First of all, the process of egg freezing itself can be stressful so anything you can do to regulate that will help. In addition, moderate exercise can help you manage the hormonal shifts that occur as a result of chronic stress. This is important because it can interfere with normal reproductive hormones required during the egg maturation process.[1303]

- **Acts as a counter to depression, and enhances mood** - When you exercise, your brain chemistry changes through the release of endorphins, which can quell anxiety[1304] [1305] and can help counter depression.[1306] [1307] Experts have even likened it to a form of meditation, giving you a sense of optimism, calmness, and clarity.[1308] All of which will support your psychological wellbeing throughout the egg freezing process. Even just going for brisk walks can help you reap many mental health and mood enhancement benefits.[1309] [1310]

- **Promotes better sleep** - Engaging in low to moderate intensity exercise can help you improve both the quality and quantity of your sleep. A meta-analytical review of 66 research studies revealed that even just one moderate workout session can increase total sleep time, reduce the time spent getting to sleep, increase overall sleep efficiency and can increase the amount of REM sleep you get at night.[1311] As you'll discover in the next chapter, a sufficient amount of good quality sleep offers a host of reproductive benefits.[1312] [1313] [1314] [1315] [1316]

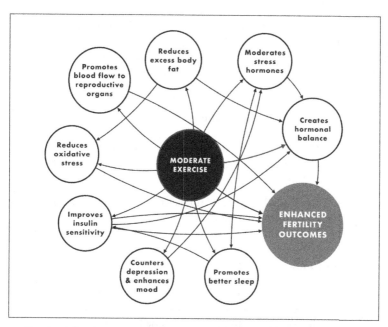

So, the scientists say that women who exercise "moderately" have the best fertility outcomes. But, what happens if exercise is a dirty word in your household? Or, on the flipside, what if you go through sneakers faster than Serena Williams - is there such a thing as getting *too much* exercise?

Well, kind of, yes: in both scenarios. Read more right below if you know you've been shirking the gym. Or, if you think you could run the risk of exercising "too much," skip down to "Team Gym Junkie " below that.

Team Couch Potato

If you consider a walk to the loo a "workout," don't worry, you're not alone: more than 77% of Americans get less than the recommended amount of exercise (2.5 hours of moderate movement each week).[1317] Here's some motivation to get Fertility Fit™: proverbial couch potatoes have a higher risk of ovulatory infertility than women who exercised 30 minutes or more a day.[1318] And the benefits are even more pronounced for women who are overweight.[1319] [1320] [1321] While it's hard to discern in particular studies if the benefits to fertility were a direct result of the exercise itself or if they were intertwined with any weight loss that may have resulted from the exercise, the research overall is clear that moderate exercise is beneficial for everyone.

Before you sign up for that hectic new bootcamp, just remember that jumping into a challenging new workout routine off-the-bat isn't the best idea either. Researchers found that heavy exercise in untrained women provokes negative changes to ovarian hormones compared to women that trained at a steadier pace.[1322] It's better to introduce exercise gradually and build up.

Key actions for couch potatoes

- Develop a moderate exercise routine in the few months prior to your egg freezing procedure - it could be beneficial for your fertility.

- Start slowly and build up the frequency, duration and intensity of your fitness routine over time - you're less likely to get injured and stress your body, and more likely to stick to it!

Team Gym Junkie

When it comes to your egg health, there is such a thing as too much of a good thing. Researchers don't know the exact reason why people who over-exercise have issues with fertility, but one hypothesis is that it generates an over-abundance of oxidative stress. Oxidative stress, as you know, is associated with impaired fertility.[1323 1324 1325 1326] What makes this complex is that exercise, by its very nature, is an oxidative process in which free radicals are generated.[1327] When you exercise moderately, your body generates adequate antioxidant defenses to protect itself.[1328] The trouble is, when you exercise to the extreme, the body can't keep up the production of these defenses to match the increasing oxidative stress.[1329 1330] The extent of which depends on the exercise duration, intensity, fitness condition and your nutritional status.

The other potential issue with over-exercise is that you may not be getting enough food energy to support both this level of exercise as well as to support your other necessary and normal functions like walking and digestion.[1331] This concept is called "energy availability," which refers to the amount of energy left over and available for your body's functions after energy has been used for training.[1332] More than thirty years of studies have shown that women who do lots of exercise without adequate nutrition and caloric energy to support it are at increased risk of reproductive problems.[1333] [1334] [1335] Energy deficiency affects fertility because important reproductive hormones stop being produced when there isn't enough available energy to sustain them. [1336] [1337] [1338] [1339] [1340] Even energy deficits garnered over one day have been shown to have adverse effects on hormone concentrations.[1341] And even one month with a large drop in energy intake could have a negative affect your reproductive hormones.[1342]

A classic example of this is women who do sports where having a low body weight or lean physique is intertwined with success. For instance, studies have found that up to 79% of ballet dancers, runners, figure skaters and gymnasts report menstrual irregularities.[1343] So, if you're exercising frequently and to the point of exhaustion, or skipping meals to slim down while continuing the same level of activity, you should be paying close attention, as you could be putting your reproductive health at risk.[1344] [1345]

Nobody is saying you should quit your sport or stop working out - professional athletes have babies all the time! However, we do know that working out to the extreme does make you more likely to experience menstrual issues. If you train and refuel responsibly, especially under the care of an expert like a coach, you are unlikely to be putting your egg freezing cycle at risk - let's get that clear. However, if you are looking to *optimize your chances*, then the studies suggest cooling off a bit in the months leading up to your procedure could do that. It's worth considering how egg freezing fits into your sports schedule and how it should be avoided while you're in a peak training period. In addition, during the actual hormonal stimulation and retrieval phase and while you recover, doctors will advise limiting movement to gentle activities.

Ways that you can over-exercise

This is a tricky question, because each person's energy metabolism is different. That said, scientists have determined the three main aspects that contribute to your fertility that can be used as guidelines for shaping your own eggxercise approach:

Frequency - if you are physically active every day of the week *and* those workouts are all intensive, you could be more than three times more likely to experience fertility problems than women who are sedentary. This is according to Norwegian researchers who studied the exercise habits and reproductive systems of nearly 4,000 women.[1346] Are you taking rest days to let your body recover?

Duration - if you exercise for over four hours a week for an extended period of time, you could be 40% less likely to have a child compared to women who don't exercise at all. And, a US study of women undergoing

IVF found that frequent exercisers were almost three times more likely to have their entire IVF cycle cancelled because their bodies didn't sufficiently respond to the treatment.[1347]

Sudden increases – The effect of exercise on your fertility is not necessarily dependent on how much you exercise, but how much you do *relative to your current ability level*.[1348] [1349] So, this is particularly relevant to those who usually exercise minimally or moderately and then suddenly take on a new challenge and radically up level their activity. Signing up for a marathon or getting an unlimited pass to Barry's Bootcamp is likely not the best way to prepare for egg freezing if you don't already regularly do them.

As you consider your exercise routine for the months leading up to your procedure, remember to take into account your nutrition habits, current body weight, existing fitness level, and overall caloric expenditure (for instance, if you have a physically active job). As a starting point, use the symptom checkers below to see if you might be over-exercising or if you have an energy deficiency, and then adjust accordingly. [1350] [1351] [1352] [1353] [1354] [1355] [1356]

SYMPTOM CHECKER: ARE YOU OVER-EXERCISING?

Low energy availability - The signs and symptoms below might be an indication from your body that you're not giving it enough energy (calories) to sustain important processes like reproduction to take place.

- ☐ Absent or irregular periods (in particular, this is linked to suppressed follicular growth, immature eggs, poor endometrial quality, spontaneous abortion and infertility)
- ☐ Chronic fatigue
- ☐ Anemia
- ☐ Recurring infections and illnesses
- ☐ Depression
- ☐ Eating disorders
- ☐ Inability to gain or build muscle or strength
- ☐ Poor athletic performance
- ☐ Stress fractures or repeated bone injuries
- ☐ Decreased muscle strength
- ☐ Irritability
- ☐ Always being hurt or injured
- ☐ Training hard but not improving performance
- ☐ Gastrointestinal problems
- ☐ Weight loss

A downloadable version of this checklist is available at elanzawellness.com.

If you checked more than two of the boxes above, ensure that you speak to your healthcare practitioner about your exercise routine as you could be potentially causing harm to your health and future fertility outcomes.

Key takeaways if you feel you are over-exercising:

- Reduce the frequency and duration of your current exercise routine.
- Avoid sudden increases in physical activity.
- Ensure that you eat sufficient, healthy calories for your level of energy expenditure.
- In particular, look out for menstrual disturbances, which are typical of people with energy deficiencies - these are linked to suppressed follicular growth, immature eggs, poor endometrial quality, spontaneous abortion and infertility.[1357]

Eggxercise action plan: Three-months prior to ovarian stimulation

During each phase of your egg freezing journey, your eggs and ovaries can be impacted by how much and what type of activity you do. At this part of the journey, we'll review the exercise considerations *leading up to* the stimulation phase. Modifications to your exercise routine during and after your procedure will be covered in "Part Three."

Exercise moderately 3-5 times per week for 30-60 mins

Moderate exercise is usually defined as a five or six out of ten in the level of effort you put in during a workout. At that level, you'll feel a noticeable increase in breathing and heart rate. You should be able to talk but not sing. You'll know you've gone out of the "moderate" range if you can only say a few words without stopping for breath.[1358]

Any exercise that increases your heart rate can improve circulation and blood flow to the ovaries. Increased circulation does not require intense exercise. In fact, sticking to low impact movements during the medication phase is essential. A sensible level is cardio for 30 minutes a day, three times a week with two, 30 minute moderate strength training sessions and additional gentle yoga, stretching or meditation.

Try embracing certain exercises

While there is limited research on exactly which types of exercise are better or worse for your egg freezing outcome, there are a few physical activities recommended by doctors because they require only moderate exertion and can be adapted to your own fitness level:

- Brisk walking
- Dancing
- Light aerobics
- Leisurely bike riding or stationary bike
- Light jogging
- Swimming
- Pilates
- Hiking
- Leisurely tennis
- Stretching
- Light elliptical
- Yoga (not including Bikram or hot yoga)

Is "fertility yoga" a real thing?
The concept has gained in popularity over the last few years. So what's the story? While, there is no medical research to date that indicates the direct impact that yoga has on egg quality or overall fertility,[1359] it's often linked to fertility-friendly effects like stress reduction, weight loss and improved circulation. Researchers have found that yoga regulates stress hormones like cortisol and adrenaline.[1360] Other findings in the Journal of Complementary and Alternative Medicine suggest that yoga improves both mood and brain chemistry by increasing levels of the "feel-good" neurotransmitters.[1361] Compared to a regular yoga class, specialist fertility or pregnancy yoga classes are more mindful of movement. There should be no strenuous torsional twists or high temperature studios, which makes it a particularly good switch if you currently go to hot yoga classes.

Avoid certain types of exercises

On the other side of the spectrum, there are some types of exercise that doctors recommend cutting back on if you currently do them.

- **Avoid activities and exercises with high heat -** There is research indicating that exposure to high heat during pregnancy can cause issues such as birth defects.[1362] So while at this stage, this is not your concern, the lack of research focused on high heat exposure during preconception has led many doctors to advise against it even if you're not pregnant. That means that you might want to consider reducing activities that involve extreme heat such as hot baths, hot tubs, hot yoga, steam rooms and saunas.

- **Minimize heavy lifting** - According to researchers, women seeking fertility treatment whose work included heavy lifting (such as nurses or interior designers) produced 14% fewer eggs than women who did not, and those that were produced were of a poorer quality. It's speculated that this could be due to the stress such repetitive physical exertion puts on the female body and its ability to reproduce.[1363] It's not just jobs that involve heavy lifting, of course. Weight training and fitness crazes like CrossFit fit into this category.[1364 1365 1366 1367 1368] If you're a gym bunny, keep active, but now is probably not the time to start pumping iron. If you have a job that requires heavy lifting, try asking for a modified work schedule during the pre-treatment period.

- **Skip the marathon and any long haul cycling trips** - Research has shown that after running a marathon, oxidative DNA damage lasts for more than a week after the race, which could be linked to immune dysfunction after exhaustive exercise.[1369 1370 1371 1372 1373]

Key takeaways

- Exercising moderately for three to five times a week for 30-60 minutes can support your reproductive functions, especially if you are overweight.

- Make sure you are consuming more than enough healthy calories offset your daily energy expenditure.

- Extreme exercise can have a negative effect on your fertility, especially if you have a low bodyweight or if you are suddenly increasing the duration, frequency or intensity of physical activity.

- Remember to run your exercise regimen past your doctor, in particular if you are very active or if you are going to start introducing physical activity after a period of being sedentary.

FERTILITY FITNESS: PREPARATION PHASE

ADD	AVOID
☐ Brisk walking	✳ Bikram or hot yoga
☐ Dancing	✳ Extreme "boot-camp"
☐ Light aerobics	✳ Weight lifting/strength training
☐ Leisurely bike riding or stationary bike	✳ Sprinting and running
☐ Light jogging	✳ Gymnastics
☐ Swimming	✳ Boxing
☐ Pilates	✳ Martial arts
☐ Hiking	✳ Any exercises that involve jumping
☐ Leisurely tennis	✳ Intense or long-haul cycling
☐ Stretching	
☐ Light elliptical	
☐ Yoga (not including Bikram or hot yoga)	

Chapter 12: Sleeping Beautifully

"There's practically no element of our lives that's not improved by getting adequate sleep."

- Arianna Huffington

Getting enough good quality sleep is important in the buildup to your egg freezing procedure because of the direct and indirect impact it can have on reproduction.[1374] You've probably read quite a lot about poor sleep affecting all sorts of things from your likelihood of developing diseases like Alzheimer's, to your productivity at work, even how long you're likely to live! We all know that feeling of being "drunk at the wheel" at our desk if we spent the night tossing and turning.[1375]

Stands to reason then that sleep disorders are linked to everything from menstrual irregularities, heightened PMS symptoms, increased time to conception, reduced likelihood of conception and increased chance of miscarriage, to lower birth weights in newborns.[1376] [1377] [1378] [1379] [1380]

As the lines between work and life blur evermore, maybe you've noticed people around you cutting caffeine, using meditation apps and proudly talking about JOMO (the joy of missing out) after they flaked on the last social gathering. Where we all used to be competing over how little sleep we needed, now the new thing is talking about how much of a priority sleep is: sleep is officially *in*. Let's hope this is not fast fashion, as in addition to other great benefits such as mental clarity, body weight management, and general health plusses, a lifestyle that involves getting sufficient sleep makes for a solid foundation for maturing healthy eggs. We're going to discuss the science of sleep, cover specifically how it could influence your egg freezing cycle outcome, and suggest how to refine your routine to help optimize your sleep cycle to give your eggs the best beneficial "beauty sleep." (Unless it's bedtime, then put this down until tomorrow...)

Are you getting enough quality sleep?

Each of us has different lifestyles and natural proclivities towards sleep that make it hard to settle on a universally optimal sleep routine for egg health. Start by asking yourself these key questions to see if you're on the right sleep track:[1381]

QUALITY SLEEP TEST	
Yes / No	Do you get between 7-9 hours of sleep each night?
Yes / No	Do you sleep at least 85% of the total time you spend in bed?
Yes / No	Do you fall asleep within 30 minutes or less?
Yes / No	Do you wake up multiples times throughout the night?
Yes / No	If you do wake up, do you normally fall back to sleep within 20 minutes or less?

If you answered "yes" to all of these, then you're in great shape. If you answered "no" to one or more of them, you're not alone. Inadequate sleep is an issue that affects more than a third of adults worldwide.[1382] Having said that, the rule of thumb is that if you're probably doing fine if you're sleeping at least 85% of the time you are in bed. You might remember sleep as being a continuous block when you were younger, but that's not actually normal for adults. It's really common to wake up at the end of every sleep cycle (a sleep cycle lasts around 90mins). Most people wake up once - even a couple of times in the night - and some don't even remember they woke up! This happens more as we age. The red flag is if you wake very frequently, sleep very lightly, or have problems falling back to sleep if you do wake in the night.

Getting enough good quality seems to be a bigger problem for women, who are more likely than men to have difficulty falling asleep[1383] and to experience sleep disorders like insomnia.[1384]

What the science says about sleep and fertility

If you suffer from a (non-apnea related) sleep disorder, a 2018 study suggests that you are more than three times as likely to experience infertility compared to women with healthy sleeping habits.[1385] Sleep apnea is a condition when your breathing stops and starts while you sleep. There is also potentially a relationship between the average number of hours you sleep per night and the average number of eggs retrieved from fertility treatment. Researchers found a trend that for every extra hour of sleep a woman got as a per night average, she had 1.5 more eggs retrieved.[1386]

The main reason scientists deem sleep so important for reproduction is that *sleep is a hormonal process*. The same area of the brain that regulates sleep-wake hormones (including melatonin and cortisol) also triggers reproductive hormones. For example, progesterone, estrogen, leptin, and follicle stimulating hormone (FSH), which are involved in processes required for egg quality, are among the hormones released during sleep. In fact, luteinizing hormone (LH) - the production of which is thought to be the event that initiates puberty - is *only* released during sleep.[1387][1388] The relationship between sleep and fertility is complex and research on the subject is surprisingly sparse.[1389] However, we can see a hormonal domino effect that is spurred by sleep-related issues. Here are examples of just a few:

Leptin - the green light for reproduction

Leptin is a key reproductive hormone that increases while you sleep. Leptin is most commonly associated with appetite, but it is also involved in key processes that rely on adequate energy balance, including reproduction. Researchers, therefore, believe it signals to the brain whether there is enough energy for reproduction to take place.[1390] In fact, leptin has even been thought to give ovaries the green light to function,[1391] and forms part of the signal that triggers ovulation to occur.[1392] The influence of leptin fluctuations on egg quality and reproductive outcomes has been identified but needs further clarification.[1393][1394][1395] What we do know is that sleep impacts the balance of leptin levels and leptin plays a central role in reproductive health.[1396]

Melatonin hormone - the ultimate egg antioxidant

Your body naturally produces melatonin, which is sometimes called "the sleepy hormone" due to its role in signaling that it's time for you to go to sleep.[1397] It is secreted when your brain perceives it's evening and stays elevated for about twelve hours throughout the night until your brain perceives dawn. For this reason, the hormone is sensitive to the cadence of your sleep patterns and could be disrupted if you sleep at different times each night, or if you try to counter nature by staying up at night and sleeping during the day (e.g. working the night shift or jet lag).

But this hormone does more than just regulate your sleep. If you think back to the "Supplementing Your Diet" chapter, we highlighted controlled studies in which it is shown that melatonin supplements can act as a uniquely potent antioxidant inside the ovaries, to neutralize harmful free radicals.[1398][1399][1400][1401][1402][1403] Because of this, egg/follicle development,[1404] the number of eggs retrieved,[1405] egg quality,[1406][1407] fertilization rates[1408] and embryonic development[1409] have all been demonstrated to be improved by melatonin.[1410][1411][1412][1413][1414] That's not to say you must take a melatonin supplement (that's up to you), but to illustrate the importance of melatonin - this key sleep hormone - for fertility. Regulating your melatonin hormone levels naturally by keeping good sleep hygiene should be a priority, whether or not you also then choose to use a supplement.

Male fertility is affected by sleep too

A 2018 study found that men who sleep five hours a night have significantly smaller testicles than those who sleep seven hours or more.[1415] And, another study found that getting less than six hours of sleep a night reduces a man's chances of getting a woman pregnant by 43%. There might be a point of diminishing returns, though, with the same study indicating that more than nine hours reduces the chances of pregnancy by a similar 42%. The optimal time is around seven hours per night.[1416]

The link between sleep and hormones such as leptin and melatonin is the primary reason that researchers think insufficient or disturbed sleep could have implications for your fertility.[1417] However, sleep is also thought to play a role in fertility in wider, indirect ways:

- **Regulates stress levels and mental health** - It used to be thought that sleep problems were a result of mental health issues, but new research indicates that sleep problems might actually be one of the *causes* of mental health issues such as depression.[1418] Studies have shown that sleep deprivation leads to changes in your brain chemistry that make it difficult for you to manage your mood and emotions,[1419] so getting good quality sleep may help you manage to fend off chronic stress that could impair fertility.[1420] Getting enough sleep will also be a game-changer during the hormonal stimulation phase when your emotions are already running high.

- **Helps maintain a fertility-friendly bodyweight** - When you don't get enough sleep, you eat more: 385 more kcal over the course of 24 hours, to be exact.[1421] If sleep deprivation is sustained, it tips the scales against you keeping a "fertility friendly" bodyweight. Sleep disorders can mean disrupted leptin levels, leading to hunger and obesity, [1422] [1423] and sleep deprivation also activates the areas in your brain associated with instant gratification and reward (and who rewards themselves with celery sticks?).[1424]

- **Modulates glucose tolerance, insulin secretion & inflammation** - In a similar vein, sleep deprivation has been shown to increase insulin resistance, which can cause reproductive hormone imbalance and contribute to weight gain.[1425] [1426] [1427] This is especially pertinent for women with

PCOS, a condition in which high levels of insulin cause the ovaries to produce more testosterone, which can then disrupt the maturation and ovulation of eggs.[1428] It also impacts women with endometriosis, as disruptions in circadian rhythm can create inflammation,[1429] which is thought to exacerbate symptoms.[1430]

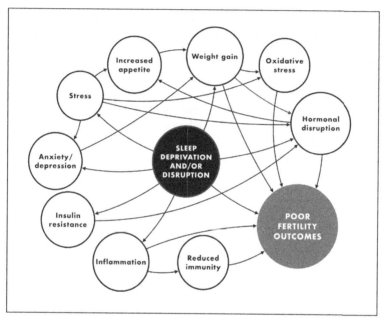

BONUS BENEFIT: Enough sleep really does make you better looking

Research from Stockholm University compared how attractive people with only five hours of sleep were rated by strangers compared to people who were allowed a full eight hours. The faces of those who scrimped on sleep were rated as looking more fatigued, less healthy and significantly less attractive, lending scientific weight to that warning to get your "beauty sleep."[1431]

12 tips for achieving optimal sleep

Start by incorporating these key actions into your pre-treatment planning so you can provide what scientists theorize is the best possible environment for your developing eggs:

1. Get 7-9 hours of sleep every night

This is probably not new information, but have you ever wondered *why*? While each person has slightly different sleep requirements, experts recommend getting this amount of sleep per night because that's how long it takes to successfully go through the four to five different stages of sleep, as each one lasts about 90-120 minutes. It's important for your body to reach and complete each stage because each one offers its own benefits that contribute to and are required for an optimally functioning brain, body and reproductive system.[1432] Getting enough sleep also ensures that all the hormones related to reproduction have enough time to be synthesized and secreted at the right levels.[1433]

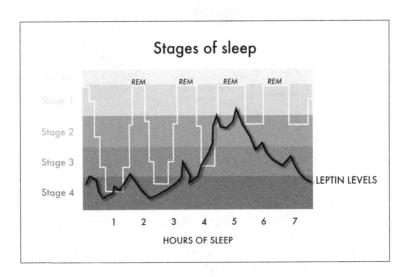

2. Work with your natural circadian rhythm

The time you go to sleep and wake up everyday helps regulate your body's circadian rhythm (the *other* biological clock). Many of your reproductive hormones use your circadian rhythm to determine if, when, and how much they should be pumping out into your bloodstream. Melatonin, cortisol, thyroid stimulating hormone (TSH), and prolactin (PRL) are all somewhat dependent on the consistency of this clock in order to serve their intended purpose.[1434]

While part of your circadian rhythm is determined by external cues such as light and dark, another part is determined by your own unique biological rhythms. This gives credence to the idea of being an "early bird" or a "night owl."[1435] Start by figuring out where you sit on this spectrum so you don't have to work against your body's natural cadence.

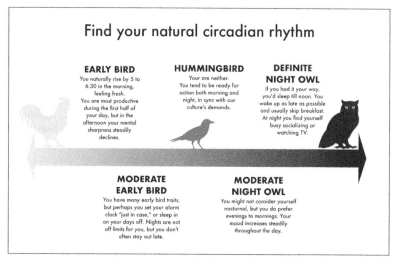

Find your natural circadian rhythm

EARLY BIRD
You naturally rise by 5 to 6:30 in the morning, feeling fresh. You are most productive during the first half of your day, but in the afternoon your mental sharpness steadily declines.

HUMMINGBIRD
Your are neither. You tend to be ready for action both morning and night, in sync with our culture's demands.

DEFINITE NIGHT OWL
If you had it your way, you'd sleep till noon. You wake up as late as possible and usually skip breakfast. At night you find yourself busy socializing or watching TV.

MODERATE EARLY BIRD
You have many early bird traits, but perhaps you set your alarm clock "just in case," or sleep in on your days off. Nights are not off limits for you, but you don't often stay out late.

MODERATE NIGHT OWL
You might not consider yourself nocturnal, but you do prefer evenings to mornings. Your mood increases steadily throughout the day.

Despite obvious limitations driven by your job and other responsibilities, optimizing your schedule and activities around your natural clock will help you fall asleep and wake up more naturally.

3. Keep consistent sleep/wake times

Because melatonin works with your innate circadian rhythm, its timing and release is very susceptible to small shifts in the sleep-wake cycle, which is why it's important to go to sleep and wake up at the same time every day.[1436]

Most of the prior research on the subject has been focused on how the erratic work and sleep schedules of nurses is associated with a higher risk of preterm birth. Building on this, a 2018 study at Washington University measured the sleep data from 176 womens' activity trackers and found that women conceived fastest if they went to bed around the same time every night. In contrast, those whose bedtime changed wildly day to day - sometimes 11pm, sometimes one o'clock in the morning - took the longest to conceive.[1437]

The best way to kickstart this habit is to focus on waking up at the same time every day, rather than the time you go to sleep. This strategy is really helpful if you have trouble getting and staying asleep throughout the night, as it actually helps build a desire to fall asleep earlier. Things to avoid are those late Sunday snoozes that can throw off your whole week. And avoid hitting the snooze button, even for a few minutes - consistency is key. If this is a struggle for you, let the sunshine in for 15 to 30 minutes right when your alarm goes off. During the winter months, try getting a light therapy box that you can put on your desk, or an alarm that gradually wakes you with light. This will help reinforce your body's circadian rhythm and might even give you an extra boost of vitamin D!

4. Sleep when it's dark

Another key to getting good sleep is to sync your circadian rhythm with your environment, including light and dark. Despite the fact that each of us might swing slightly on the earlier or late side, darkness is nature's way of putting us to sleep. If you've ever experienced jetlag, you can attest to how awful it is when these two forces are fighting against each other!

The importance of sleeping while it's dark outside can be illustrated in studies conducted on shift workers who sleep during the day and work at night. Because melatonin levels rise when it's dark outside, it makes sense why their melatonin patterns were irregular. This translated to higher rates of infertility[1438] [1439] and upwards of 28% fewer eggs retrieved in an IVF cycle compared to women who slept during normal hours.[1440]

It's obviously impossible to avoid in some cases - such as for cabin crew and some doctors and nurses - but if you have some say in your shift rotation, then the research indicates that avoiding unsociable working hours as much as is possible during the three months could be worth the effort, as working the night shift is linked to fertility problems.[1441]

5. Spend time in the sun during the day

Just as darkness indicates that it's time to sleep, spending time in the sun can be just as beneficial, showing your body when it's *not* time to sleep. Studies show that exposure to bright daylight can significantly increase melatonin production at night by regulating your circadian rhythm.[1442] [1443] [1444] Getting this daily dose of natural vitamin D can enhance both your sleep quality and duration, especially if you suffer from insomnia.[1445] [1446] [1447]

6. "Sleep-ify" your bedroom

- **Reduce exposure to outside noise** - This means sudden, startling, loud or unexpected sounds, e.g. traffic horns or barking dogs, which are linked to poor quality sleep.[1448] [1449] [1450] [1451] Try earplugs or sleeping with a white noise track playing in the background. Investing in some heavy curtains can help create a sound barrier.

- **Consider some soothing sounds** - Rhythmic sounds have the opposite effect and can be soporific, helping you to relax while you're getting ready for bed. Switch them off before you actually fall asleep though, as some research suggests some auditory tones could disrupt sleep if they chime at different times to your own brainwaves.

- **Keep your bedroom between 60° - 70°F (16° - 21°C)** - Studies show that if your room or body temperature is too cold or too warm, you might have a hard time falling asleep, staying asleep throughout the night,[1452] [1453] [1454] [1455] or just in general getting quality sleep. Try setting your thermostat to a pleasant 65°F, which is thought to be optimal for the "average" person. Heat regulation is less efficient when you are in deep sleep. Wear loose, breathable clothing made of comfortable fabric so you can help maintain an optimal body temperature as the air temperature fluctuates throughout the night.[1456]

- **Use dim red lights for night lights** - Red light has the least power to shift circadian rhythm and suppress melatonin.[1457] Blue light has the strongest ability to reset our own circadian rhythm, which is why it should be avoided for at least a few hours before bed.[1458]

- **Firm up your mattress** - A medium-firm mattress has been shown to positively affect sleep quality and prevent sleep disturbances and muscular discomfort [1459] [1460]

- **Try an orthopedic pillow** - One study measured the sleep patterns among orthopedic, feather and memory foam pillows and found that orthopedics are the best for your neck curve, temperature and comfort, which could affect sleep quality.[1461]

- **Test out a weighted blanket** - If you have trouble letting go of the day and "settling" before sleep, a weighted blanket could help you unwind and increase sleep duration and quality, according to a 2015 study.[1462]

- **Get blackout blinds** - If your bedroom is exposed to natural or synthetic light when you want to be sleeping, getting extra thick blackout blinds can be a great way to get your natural melatonin flowing.

7. Try to de-stress before bed

Oftentimes anxiety and stress are accompanied by a variety of sleep issues such as difficulty falling asleep, trouble staying asleep, waking up early, overall poor quality sleep and even more severe disorders like insomnia.[1463] [1464] When stress and anxiety are present, they activate the adrenaline, cortisol and norepinephrine hormones, which are responsible for boosting energy, alertness and heart rate (needed to keep you alive in a "fight or flight" scenario). As you can imagine, these are counterproductive to achieving a peaceful night's sleep.[1465] Try adding some of these simple activities to your pre-bedtime routine.

- **Try relaxation techniques like breathing and meditation** - The "relaxation response" has been proposed by scientists as a way to counter the "stress response."[1466] Deep, slow, self-aware breathing is an ancient and powerful way to clear the body of stress and tension, and a great way to relax as part of a nightly transition to sleep. There are lots of apps on the market that can help you unwind.

- **Get a massage** - As if you need an excuse for this one... but gentle massage has been shown to improve sleep quality in people who are ill.[1467] The release of oxytocin, serotonin and dopamine can be released during sessions, which can foster feelings of calmness and connectedness and could potentially counter the effects of cortisol and adrenaline.[1468] If you can't afford to splurge after paying out for treatment, how about asking a friend or partner if they'll do the honors? TIP: during the hormonal stimulation phase, stick to massages that avoid your abdomen or the center of your body, which might be swollen or uncomfortable.

8. Don't use electronic devices such as cell phones, computers and televisions two hours before bedtime

The blue, dawn-like light from these screens has been found to increase the risk of sleep disorders. Even dim light can interfere with your circadian rhythm and melatonin secretion.[1469] [1470] [1471] [1472] Not only that, but people often associate using laptops with work stress, which can get your mind whirring all over again. The point is not to avoid activities in the evening - it's to choose activities that are mentally soothing or relaxing rather than mentally stimulating. If you struggle to go to sleep right away when you go to bed, instead try reading a book, listening to a podcast or a meditation track.

9. Avoid alcohol

You might think that alcohol might actually *help* you get to sleep, but new research reveals that even as little as one alcoholic drink can impair the restorative quality of sleep by more than nine percent. Moderate alcohol consumption lowers restorative sleep quality by 24%, and high alcohol intake by as much as 39%.[1473] So, even if you get more hours of sleep, chances are it will be super low quality.

10. Don't drink lots of liquid before bed

This one's pretty simple – if you drink a lot you're more likely to wake up and use the bathroom! Stay hydrated throughout the day, for sure, but try not to drink too much one to two hours before bed.

11. Don't drink lots of caffeinated drinks during the day

Research has shown that drinking excessive amounts of coffee or other caffeinated beverages even during the day can throw off your circadian rhythm[1474] and can decrease your melatonin production over time.[1475] [1476] One or two cups is fine but try to drink them more than eight hours before bedtime.

12. Don't smoke

Yet another reason to quit! Studies have shown that cigarette smokers are significantly more likely than non-smokers to have problems going to sleep, staying asleep and being sleepy during the day, and they have higher daily caffeine intake.[1477] [1478] High doses of nicotine have a stimulant effect, which will also make it harder to get to sleep in the first place.

What about CBD oil?

Research on CBD oil and sleep is in its infancy and has yielded mixed results. At present, there just isn't enough data to merit a definitive viewpoint. Remember, in many states (and other countries) it is illegal.

Key takeaways:

- Sleep is a hormonal process and, as such, getting too little or only bad quality sleep could significantly impact your egg freezing outcome.

- Sleep-linked hormones such as melatonin and leptin play a crucial role in fertility. The pattern and release of these hormones are partly dependent on sleep timing, duration and quality.

CHECKLIST: SLEEP OPTIMIZATION

Actions

- [ ] Get 7-9 hours of sleep every night
- [ ] Find your natural circadian rhythm
- [ ] Keep a consistent sleep/wake schedule
- [ ] Sleep when it's dark out and avoid working the night shift
- [ ] Spend time in the sun during the day
- [ ] Take a warm bath or shower 90 min before bed
- [ ] Try relaxation techniques like deep breathing and meditation before bed
- [ ] Get a massage before bed
- [ ] Don't drink alcohol
- [ ] Don't smoke
- [ ] Don't drink lots of liquid before bed
- [ ] Don't drink lots of coffee or caffeinated beverages throughout the day, especially near bedtime
- [ ] Use electronic devices such as cell phones, computers and televisions two hours before bedtime

Tips to "sleep-ify" your bedroom

- [ ] Reduce outside noise
- [ ] Keep your bedroom between 60 - 70°F (15 - 20°C)
- [ ] Use dim red lights for night lights
- [ ] Install blackout blinds
- [ ] Invest in a medium firm mattress
- [ ] Get an orthopedic pillow
- [ ] Test out a weighted blanket
- [ ] Get an artificial light for an alarm

A downloadable version of this checklist is available at
ELANZAwellness.com.

BONUS CHAPTER: Let's Talk About Stress

"Remember that stress doesn't come from what's going on in your life. It comes from your thoughts about what's going on in your life."

- Andrew J. Bernstein

For two things that are so often mentioned in the same sentence, there are surprisingly few firm findings about the relationship between stress and fertility. It's absolutely clear that women with infertility have higher levels of anxiety and depression, so scientists know that infertility causes stress (duh). Preliminary studies also appear to have found the biological link that explains how chronic stress can impact the reproductive system, but more research into those exact mechanisms are needed before we understand this fully.

Regardless, it's not good for your overall health to be stressed. We all know that the words "don't stress" can sometimes just get you *more* stressed about having stress (and how that could affect your treatment), so we're not here to tell you to quit your high powered job or stop taking on so many challenges. Instead, this section is simply here to give you a more scientific understanding of what the mechanisms behind stress actually are, how scientists think they could be linked with your reproductive system and how you can better manage the stresses that life will ultimately entail. It's wild how even a few tools that help you proactively manage stressful situations can transform the way you feel about your day and your life and give you some peace of mind that will ideally make the whole egg freezing process more enjoyable...and possibly more fruitful.

You've almost certainly heard stories about couples struggling with "unexplained infertility," whose lives revolve around the anxious pursuit of parenthood, who end up throwing in the towel on stressful treatments, only to find out they're pregnant naturally. Or, how about those couples who decide to give up on fertility treatments and adopt, only to find out they're pregnant a couple of months later?[1479] These anecdotes are almost always chalked up to the influence of stress "switching off" fertility. For this reason, amongst others, stress is the number one lifestyle question fertility doctors tell us they get asked by their patients.

Despite the intuitive connection, the finer details of the relationship between stress and fertility are not yet fully understood.[1480] [1481] [1482] [1483] Studies on the subject are mostly centered on infertile couples, making it hard to determine whether infertile people are stressed because they're coping with infertility, or if they are infertile because they are stressed, or both.[1484][1485][1486] Even despite the biological plausibility of stress hormones such as cortisol and adrenaline potentially disrupting your reproductive hormones, there is no consensus that stress will have any dramatic effect on the outcome of your fertility treatment.[1487]

DOCTOR PERSPECTIVE: "Despite my advice against it, I had one patient quit her job because she was so worried about how stress would impact her IVF cycle. It did not impact the outcome of the cycle. However, I do think she was happy to get a new job!" - Dr. Carolyn Givens, Pacific Fertility Center, San Francisco

Not all stress is created equal

Stress is quite a broad-reaching term that is used loosely, but actually manifests itself in different ways, biologically. It exists in two forms: acute (reacting to immediate, life-threatening danger) and chronic (acute stresses experienced consistently over time).

When you encounter something your subconscious perceives as a threat, the "fight or flight" chain reaction kicks in, a reaction that is hardwired into your body in order to increase your chances of immediate survival.[1488][1489][1490][1491][1492][1493] That's a good thing. That powerful surge of adrenaline is what keeps you alive when you almost step in front of a moving car, or helps you duck when something heavy flies towards your head. That's acute stress. In an acutely stressful situation, once the threat disappears, your adrenaline level will drop back to normal.

However, if your body is kept continually in a state that it perceives as stressful (like if you're deeply worried about your ticking biological clock, or worried about paying your bills...!) and it you don't know how to "throw yourself a bone" and properly deactivate and manage these stressful thoughts and feelings, the stress can become *chronic*. And the effects of chronic stress on fertility, specifically for women, has been shown to persist long after the stress is gone.[1494] Chronic stress is what doctors refer to when they suggest patients "de-stress," not things like avoiding scary movies or roller coasters. Our hectic, over-stimulated lives, jacked-up, tired and wired on caffeine and electronics, are a recipe for exhaustion and leave us wide open to existing in a permanent state of (chronic) physically-felt stress.

Chronic stress can be mitigated with mind-related self-care (which we'll outline below), but the good news is that by following many of the other tenants of your egg health regimen, you'll be helping your body cope with the biological impact of stress too!

DOCTOR PERSPECTIVE: "We know that chronic stress has a physical effect on reproductive organs, but managing the mental emotional aspects of stress can be challenging and can affect everyone differently. Even if you don't consider yourself someone who is chronically stressed, adapting healthy lifestyle choices can help mitigate any oxidative stress that is happening on a cellular level. When patients are going through the egg freezing process I emphasize self care techniques such as massages, avoiding/limiting alcohol and making sure they are getting plenty of rest." -
Dr. Hemalee Patel, Lifestyle Medicine Expert, San Francisco

What the science says about stress and fertility

When you're chronically stressed, cortisol does not return to normal. When it stays elevated, it causes a hormonal chain reaction that affects everything from your nervous and immune systems to your metabolism (you also have cortisol to thank for stubborn belly fat[1495]) to your reproductive system.[1496 1497 1498] Hormonal balance plays a role in reproduction,[1499] which is why chronic stress is thought to interfere with normal follicle development,[1500] menstruation,[1501 1502 1503] ovulation,[1504] live birth rates,[1505] fewer eggs retrieved, egg maturation,[1506] reduced fertilization rates[1507 1508] and longer time to pregnancy.[1509 1510 1511 1512]

A team of neuroendocrinology researchers from the University of Otago in New Zealand claim to have run studies that prove that fertility is suppressed during times of chronic stress.[1513] Here's what they found:

- A group of nerve cells near the base of the brain – called RFRP neurons – suppress the reproductive system during periods of chronic stress.

- When the activity of the RFRP cells is increased due to the stress hormone cortisol, reproductive hormoes are disrupted.

- Hormones functioned normally when the RFRP neurons were silenced, even when in stressful situations.

"RFRP neurons are a critical piece of the puzzle in stress-induced suppression of reproduction," according to Professor Greg Anderson, who led the research. "These neurons become active in stressful situations – perhaps by sensing the increasing levels of cortisol – and they then suppress the reproductive system." Based on this research, here's what you need to know:

- High levels of stress hormone (cortisol) can trigger a chain reaction in your body that suppresses fertility.

- Practicing calming proven techniques to reduce chronic stress and anxiety could be beneficial for reproductive outcomes.

- In the future, new drugs to block the actions of the RFRP neurons may be developed to help women struggling with infertility.

DOCTOR PERSPECTIVE: "We all have stress! It is impossible to eliminate completely. We don't know the true impact of stress on fertility, but thankfully it plays a very minor role, if any. I recommend findings ways to MANAGE stress - whether it is exercise, mindfulness, or therapy. It will help women have a more positive experience with their cycle, as well as help in other aspects of their life!" - Dr. Meera Shah, Nova IVF, Mountain View

Getting stress in check

Whatever your lifestyle or whatever you're facing, getting stress in check is less about making radical changes and more about making subtle alterations to your mindset and daily routine. Sometimes it's about perception, not perfection. When we face adverse events or experiences according to our own perception, our bodies can be stimulated to produce stress hormones that trigger a 'flight or fight' response and activate our immune system.[1514] So what can you do to change your mindset and your coping mechanisms?

- **Develop an "optimistic" mindset** - This sounds hard, but it is possible because your thoughts are pretty freaking powerful. Creating some positive mantras is a good way to begin. Focus on the solution (egg freezing), rather than the problem. You're reading this, you're being proactive. You are right in your power right now!

- **Exercise in moderation** - As well as the physiological benefits we covered earlier, moderate exercise is an absolutely *fantastic* way to let off steam and ease stress. It might feel like a pain to pull on your leggings and head out the door, but it's so worth it: just think of those glorious endorphins you're going to feel rushing through you.

- **Meditate** - Give conscious breathing techniques or a guided meditation podcast a whirl if stillness doesn't come easily to you. Worth a shot, right?

- **Try acupuncture** - This ancient practice involves placing slender needles into various pressure points on the body. While the research is still preliminary, there's some indication that it can help manage the perception of stress.[1515] In fact, many clinics recommend it for couples going through infertility treatment, whether there's some direct benefit to male and female fertility or if it's rather a way to help them manage the stress of infertility, it is the most embraced alternative medicine in the fertility community.

DOCTOR INSIGHT: "There is growing evidence that acupuncture is beneficial to help alleviate stress, decrease pain and aid fertility. Egg freezing and fertility in general tends to be a stressful, anxiety provoking conversation to have. In my opinion, when a patient comes to me to ask my thoughts regarding acupuncture and optimizing fertility I discuss/review the literature, latest research and science with them and am happy to incorporate it as a modality to be used in conjunction with the other treatment options. Using this type of integrative, multidisciplinary approach gives patients more control. On the whole, I see more potential upsides than I do downsides." - Dr. Hemalee Patel, Lifestyle Medicine Expert, San Francisco

- **Laugh more** - Laughter can reduce the physical effects of stress (like fatigue) on the body. Our brains are reciprocally interconnected with our emotions and facial expressions - if you're frowning, you feel worse. If you smile, you'll feel happier. It's not a one way street. When people are stressed, they often hold a lot of the stress in their face. So laughing or smiling can help relieve some of that tension and improve the situation.[1516] [1517] [1518] In fact, according to a Harvard study, a total of just 20 minutes a day of laughter or play can decrease stress symptoms by up to 50%.[1519] Buy some tickets to a stand-up show or put on your favorite old comedy movie.

- **Journal** - Keeping a journal may be one way to effectively relieve stress-related symptoms due to its meditative and reflective effects [1520] [1521] A gratitude journal, in particular, can really help put things in perspective. Just pick a time every day to write down a few things that make you happy.

- **Find a support network** - A problem shared is a problem halved. Pick carefully though. If your sister is a stress trigger, for instance, it may not do much to alleviate your stress if you try to share your work woes with her.[1522] Surround yourself with caring, positive people who enrich your life.

- **Hug your stress away** - Hugging may actually reduce blood pressure and stress levels in adults.[1523] Alternatively, book a massage for the same power of touch benefits.

- **Get creative** - Research shows that art therapy can potentially reduce stress-related behavior and symptoms.[1524]

- **Listen to music** - If you are feeling stressed or are anticipating a stressful event, research indicates that music triggers biochemical stress reducers, which can help alleviate the situation.[1525] [1526] This might also help your brain develop a more positive association to the stress trigger, reducing its impact in the future.

- **Therapy** - Turns out something as simple as lying on the couch might be the ticket to better fertility! Research into therapy's potential positive impacts on fertility are promising. In particular, Cognitive Behavioral Therapy (CBT, in which patients are taught to turn negative thoughts into positive ones) shows good results. Women receiving CBT have shown results such as improved rates of conception in IVF[1527] [1528] [1529] [1530] and ESHRE even suggests that behavioral therapy can restore ovulation in infertile women.[1531] Cognitive therapy for stress rests on the premise that it's not only the events in our lives that make us stressed, it's the way we think about them - you have the power to filter and change how you experience events. No one method of therapy works for everyone one - try group support or more straight-up talking therapy if that's more your bag.

PART TWO Summary: Putting it all into action

We've covered a lot of "fertile" ground (couldn't help ourselves, sorry) in this Preparing Your Eggs For Freezing section: we detailed how and what to eat to optimize fertility, supplements to consider, getting the balance right with exercise, refining your sleep practices and, finally, starting to de-stress your way towards fertility fitness.

It may feel overwhelming to take on all these small changes at once, especially if you're burning the candle at both ends like a lot of us these days! We find that a winning strategy is to identify a few key areas of focus, whether that's getting your blood sugar in check and/or replacing your kitchen and bathroom products with fertility-friendly ones, and, as a super easy minimum, adding a few key supplements to your daily routine. Take it one area at a time, at your pace. Just remember that every action brings you one step forward towards setting the best conditions for optimal egg health. And the benefits don't stop there: think of each bit of effort you make as a renovation of your overall reproductive health that could have benefits for years to come.

To help keep your fertility fitness on track, you can visit our website, which we'll be updating with all kinds of useful tips, resources, stories, up-to-date information and our own personal spin on things. We want your egg freezing journey to be as positive and empowering as possible, so consider this an open invitation for you to get in touch and share your own journey...we can't wait to hear how you get on.

Right now, or whenever you're ready, move on to Part Three: Owning Your Procedure, to dive right down into the nuts and bolts of what we're all here for, the retrieval procedure itself!

PART THREE: OWNING YOUR PROCEDURE

Your stimulation cycle go-to guide

"I have learned over the years that when one's mind is made up, this diminishes fear; knowing what must be done does away with fear."

— *Rosa Parks*

You're on the home stretch of your egg freezing journey! Part Three of this guide is your companion through all the stages of the actual treatment and beyond: from pre-injection mental and practical preparations, to how you might feel throughout the stimulation cycle, to what your next steps might be after your retrieval. You could read this chapter all in one go, then also refer back to particular sections at the relevant time during your treatment cycle for a quick refresher.

Before your stimulation cycle begins

Setup your schedule
Plan your prescription procurement
Clear up any unknowns
Anticipate lifestyle modifications
Prepare emotionally
Establish a support system
Create a positive mindset routine

What to expect day-by-day throughout ovarian stimulation

DAY 1: Injections begin
DAYS 2 - 6
DAYS 7 - 9
DAY 10: The "trigger shot"
DAY 11: Retrieval day prep
DAY 12: Retrieval day
DAY 13+: Recovery

The future - "What should I do now?"

If you got the results you wanted
If the results weren't what you wanted
Ongoing storage of your eggs
Using your frozen eggs: if you struggle to conceive naturally
Looking forward: fertility treatments are improving by the day
What else can you do?

Chapter 14: Before Your Stimulation Cycle Begins

"Only someone who is well prepared has the opportunity to improvise."

— *Ingmar Bergman*

First, let's look at the *practical* schedule and life preparations for your EF cycle. Knowing what's to come and planning accordingly can be liberating and help give you a smoother ride throughout the course of treatment. Despite this, no one can predict exactly how the cycle is going to unfold for you: every woman's egg freezing cycle follows a slightly different timeline, duration and outcome. When you head into an egg freezing cycle, you're just going to have to expect the unexpected to a certain degree.

1. Setup your schedule to factor in two weeks of appointments, retrieval and recovery

The average egg freezing cycle takes 12 days. That's from the first day of hormone injections (which usually start two to three days after you get your period) right up until the retrieval procedure. However, the exact duration will depend on how your ovaries respond to the injections. If the cycle takes more or less time than this, it doesn't mean anything is wrong, it just means your ovaries are responding to the hormones at their own pace. Timing can be affected by age and medical conditions, such as PCOS.

TIP: You can ask your doctor in advance how long they anticipate your cycle taking, but remember, it's just an educated guesstimate and your body will work to its own timesheet!

Try to maintain a flexible schedule

During the treatment cycle, you'll need to visit the clinic anywhere from four to eight times for your doctor to monitor the growth of your follicles and adjust your fertility medications.

At the start, the clinic can give you a rough idea of when those appointments are likely to be, but they may change depending how your ovaries are responding. Because you won't know for sure when you'll need to go in, you should avoid making any travel plans over the stimulation phase and recovery period.

TIP: Before the start of your cycle, ask the clinic if there's a window of time during the day that they will conduct the scans. Block out that window of time (plus travel time to get to the clinic) in your calendar starting on at least "Day 4" from when you start the injections. This will help remind you not to schedule any important meetings over that time.

Plan on taking at least one day off work

On average, this is on Day 12 of the egg freezing cycle. But, yours could be sooner or later than that. Your egg retrieval procedure will not be scheduled ahead of time, as the exact day is subject to the doctor seeing the right amount of follicle growth on your scans.

You'll need to take the day off work for the procedure - the morning for the procedure and the afternoon to rest and recover. Most doctors say their patients are back at work the day after treatment, but that may not be the case for everyone. Anecdotally speaking, women who had an above average number of eggs retrieved (which is typical for women with PCOS and younger women) seem to take slightly longer to recover than average. That may be because the ovaries tend to be more swollen.

TIP: If your doctor tells you that you're likely to be a "good responder" and generate many eggs, you might want to anticipate an extra day off for recovery because your ovaries might be particularly swollen.

2. Plan your prescription procurement

Your clinic will help guide you through the best available options for purchasing your medications in the area, but here's a quick rundown on what you can expect and a few tips on how to streamline the process.

- **Will insurance cover any or part of the costs?** Check if your health insurance covers all or part of the medication and, if so, if they require you to use specific pharmacies or protocols.

- **Which pharmacies stock the meds?** There are only a handful of fertility specialty pharmacies that will be able to fulfill your prescription. Start by requesting a list of recommended pharmacies that stock fertility medications from your clinic.

- **What's the price?** Save money by researching different pharmacies and delivery options. It's worth shopping around a little as medications really do differ in price based on the pharmacy.

- **How will I get the meds?** In the US, most pharmacies can overnight your medications to you via FedEx or UPS. Because these medications need to be refrigerated, they are most often delivered in unmarked, Styrofoam coolers with cooler packs to keep them cold. You can receive them at home or work but make sure to keep them inside the cooler until they can be moved to a refrigerator (not the freezer!). You'll also need to be available so you can sign for the package upon delivery. If the medications cannot be delivered, you'll need to figure out where the pharmacy is and how to pick them up in accordance with your schedule. Most pharmacies will give you the medications in an indiscreet cooler bag. Just make sure to transfer the medications to a refrigerator as soon as you can.

- **How do I feel about injecting the meds?** When it comes to actually injecting the medications, many clinics offer either a one-time group class or a private instruction with a nurse to demonstrate and practice how to use them properly. Try to do this as closely as you can to the start of your treatment so it's fresh in your mind. Don't be shy about asking questions, or to have them repeat the process or even to take your own video. If you're feeling less than thrilled about injecting these hormones, we'll discuss some strategies on how to approach this in the next chapter.

- **What if you don't want to do your own injections?** Recruit a friend, co-worker, partner or family member to help - it can make a big difference to not have to press the button yourself. Just remember that this person would need to be available when the shots should be administered, and they need to be taken at the same time every day, similar to birth control pills. Hormones love a schedule! Alternatively, ask your clinic if there is a "concierge" nurse in your area who can pop over to your home to help you, for a fee.

3. Clear up any unknowns

Being aware and prepared is a sure fire way to bolster your confidence. If you ever feel like there's something you're not sure about or that you've forgotten, do not be embarrassed to ask. There are always some "known unknowns," like how many eggs you'll retrieve and the exact retrieval day. But, remember that your doctor and medical team are there to provide answers, so you should never feel embarrassed to ask questions, no matter how many of them you have. If you have any outstanding questions after leaving the clinic, call back and ask. Not only does removing the unknown help keep anxiety levels down, but also double-checking questions about medication, dosages etc. can help prevent mistakes from happening. This is your money, your procedure and your body. It's your right to make sure you're clear about what's happening and why.

"On the first day of shots, my mind completely blanked and I couldn't remember what the nurse told me about how to inject the medications… I was so embarrassed to have to call them to ask to run through it again, but I felt so much better when I did" - Liz, 27

"I felt really rushed during my monitoring appointments. I had lots of questions, but felt rude to keep asking them. The doctor was nice and he did ask me if I understood everything. In the end I found myself just saying 'yes' and then kicking myself later for not just being upfront and asking for more time." - Kira, 38

4. Anticipate lifestyle modifications

As you gear up for your stimulation cycle to begin, there are some important things you can do to prepare your body and take the pressure off your calendar (and yourself!) Most of the lifestyle modifications from Part Two still apply, but there are some added nuances that are specific to the stimulation phase that you'll want to take note of:

Diet

- Make your life a lot easier by stocking up on the right foods and healthy snacks beforehand so you don't have to worry about it.

- If there are any snacks you love, stock up on a few healthy versions of them for the latter part of the injection phase - easing up a little from your preparation nutrition guidelines won't hurt at this point and some women say they get cravings (especially towards the end of the cycle when they're staying home more.)

- Avoid stimulants. Too much caffeine, for instance, can heighten emotions. But if it makes you more emotional to NOT drink coffee, consume caffeine in moderation.

- You may not respond well to alcohol on top of the fertility drugs. Some say it left them feeling miserable. So, if you're going to drink, the keyword here is *moderation*.

- You might be feeling bloated, especially in the few days preceding your retrieval, so try to cut down on salty foods that cause water retention.

- Drink plenty of water to help flush out any bloating.

Supplements & oils

- There is no scientific evidence indicating that the supplements mentioned in the "Supplementing your Diet" chapter will interfere with the stimulation hormones. Regardless, flag them with your doctor (as well as any other supplements you might take) in case she or he advises you to discontinue them during the hormone stimulation phase.

- Consider taking a probiotic (namely, Lactobacillus acidophilus) during the stimulation phase and for a few weeks after your retrieval surgery. While the procedure is safe, there is a risk of infection.

- Aromatherapy can be a great way to de-stress, but there are some aromatherapy treatments or oils that are thought to have the potential to interfere with your hormones. It's unknown how big an impact this could have on your treatment, if any, but it's wise to avoid the following essential oils, just in case: rose, basil, clary sage, and juniper berry.

- Avoid St Johns' Wort supplements (note, these could cause birth control pills to be less effective, too)

- Avoid other herbal supplements. Hormones are complex and it's just not fully known how herbs interact with this delicate system.

DOCTOR PERSPECTIVE: "Unless specifically done to improve egg quality, it's best to cease using any herbs and supplements you are currently taking." - Dr. Paul C. Lin, Seattle Reproductive Medicine, 2019-2020 SART President

Exercise

- You might not feel like being super active but it shouldn't stop you from enjoying light exercise like a walk or less strenuous, meditative forms of yoga.

- Most important, you should avoid lifting heavy weights, contact sports and torsional twists. The doctors on our panel advise that you should avoid these activities until your next period, which usually arrives about 12-14 days after the retrieval.

Sex

There's no evidence indicating that having sex could hurt you (or your eggs!) during an ovarian stimulation cycle. Hanky-panky during the phase when you're injecting hormones initially is considered fine, as long as you use protection, e.g. a condom. If ovulation was to occur unexpectedly and you didn't use protection, you might be subject to not just one but multiple pregnancies, e.g. twins, triplets, or more. After all, the whole point of the drugs is to make you hyper-fertile and get your ovaries to mature a whole lot of eggs. Using protection after retrieval is also important because of the possibility that some eggs could be missed and not collected during the retrieval procedure. Because sperm lives in the body for up to five days, this can increase the chance of an unintended pregnancy. Doctors usually advise you to avoid having sexual intercourse after you've administered the "trigger" shot, right before your retrieval. This shot triggers the final step in maturation. You would probably find it uncomfortable anyway, as your ovaries will be enlarged. In general, the doctors we spoke to say listen to your body and be aware that intercourse can exacerbate pelvic discomfort from bloating.

DOCTOR PERSPECTIVE: "Sex during stimulation is ok as long as it's with a condom. Women also need to be aware of the risk of ovarian torsion. So, it should be "gentle" sex. I also tell my patients to avoid sex for at least 12 days after the retrieval." - Dr. Diana Chavkin, HRC Fertility, Los Angeles

5. Prepare emotionally

One of the questions women most frequently ask us is: "how are the hormones going to make me feel emotionally?" As with anything involving people and hormones, there's no single answer. But we spoke to many women undergoing egg freezing, or who had already done it, and this is what they had to say:

"I'm a bit nervous about it right now. Starting the injections is daunting and I feel a little alone. My sister, God bless her, is coming with me to the hospital for the actual surgery." - Dee, 35

It's really natural to feel some anxiety before a medical procedure. The stimulation cycle poses all kinds of new challenges, from injecting hormones to constantly reworking your schedule to accommodate the monitoring appointments. There are a lot of moving parts.

"I was filled with all kinds of self-doubt, despite having been really sure I wanted to freeze my eggs. It was like I was scanning all my past decisions that had led me to this point: was my breakup the right thing? Am I behind all my friends? Have I ever even thought if I actually want kids?" - Ellie, 34

Your plans and dreams are suddenly at the forefront; your relationships come under the spotlight. (There's nothing like paying a ton of money for something to focus your mind and crystallize your emotions!) Everything from anger, reflection, stigma, sadness, aloneness and regret has been cited as feelings noted when reflecting on what might have led to this moment.

"I nearly bit my housemate's head off for leaving a dirty dish in the sink. Even the smallest things started to really niggle me. I had to apologize to a few people after I realized how irrational I was being. Thankfully, I had told most of my close friends and family beforehand and they understood." - Julia, 33

Many women say the emotional sensitivity during the second half of the stimulation cycle is like an enhanced version of their usual symptoms of

PMS. So, if you normally find yourself easily irritated or angry, or teary and catastrophizing, or even introverted and nervous just before your period, then chances are this could be something to expect during your egg freezing cycle. On the other hand, many women don't report having any emotional fluctuations at all! In fact, some of them reported having positive emotions that highlighted their own feelings of relief and empowerment afforded by the procedure itself.

"I feel like I was anticipating the worst case scenario, emotionally. And maybe I'm just lucky, but I didn't have any anxiety or emotional ups and downs that I thought I would. Having to do the injections was a very small price to pay compared to the enormous sense of relief I have about preserving my fertility even though I don't want to have a baby right now."
- Cherise, 38

DOCTOR PERSPECTIVE: "While some underlying emotions may be enhanced, I have NEVER once had a patient stop the process prior to egg retrieval because they could not handle the emotional aspects of it. And, when I see patients back for the first ultrasound after starting stimulation the most common comment I hear is that the injections are not as difficult as they feared. And I generally hear that the experience was not as bad as they read about beforehand and that they were very happy they did it." -
Dr. Carolyn Givens, Pacific Fertility Center, San Francisco

It's particularly important to get into a good headspace emotionally in advance if your doctor has indicated you might not yield many eggs ("poor responder" is the rather awful medical term for it). Your age, and/or your test results will give the best indication of this. Research shows that women are more likely to have regrets about going through with the procedure if the cycle yields ten eggs or fewer, so you should carefully consider your doctor's prediction and make sure you only go through the cycle once you've reflected on how you'd feel if you got far fewer eggs than you want - or no eggs. It does happen. Getting very few eggs can also lead to anxiety, distress and depression, so make sure you have the right support around you - hope for the best, plan for the worst.

6. Establish a support system

Research shows that having a good support system can help reduce psychological stress (anxiety, restlessness) as well as physical stress (cortisol levels)[1532] and can even facilitate a better physical recovery.[1533] [1534] [1535] In fact, the European Society of Human Reproduction Embryology

(ESHRE) values emotional wellbeing so highly as a factor in treatment that it recommends that psychosocial support should be part of standard protocol for all types of fertility treatments.[1536] And, some research has found that people with social support after surgery recover faster.[1537]

Having the right emotional support in place during your treatment cycle could also help prevent you from having regrets, according to a study. When the researchers from this study spoke to women two years after their egg freezing treatments, they found that those who lacked emotional support and information during their procedure were more likely to have regrets about doing it in the first place.[1538] Consciously setting up a support system might entail specifically asking friends or family to help you with certain chores, to come to appointments with you or to cut you some slack if you're a little hard to live with for a couple of weeks. Maybe you just arrange a time to sit down with loved ones and talk to them about what you're doing and why you're doing it.

Opening up to family and friends about egg freezing also gives you a chance to answer any questions *they* have. It's natural for people to be curious. Some people might just come right out with it, but others will hold back, trying to respect your privacy. Educating others, be they in your immediate circle or strangers, can help you take control of your situation and remind you of why you made this empowering choice in the first place. You might be surprised to find how sharing this personal experience with family and friends could bring you closer together - a neat unexpected side effect that a lot of people have raised.

That said, knowing who to get support from and how to ask them for it might present its own anxiety. We've asked other women who froze their eggs who and how they went about shaping up a support system during treatment. Perhaps one of their stories will strike a chord with you:

"Sitting in a waiting room with a bunch of married couples, I became quite resentful of them and their smug coupledom and their joint incomes to pay for this. And then later I felt guilty for thinking that – we were all in the same sh*tty situation. Maybe their journey was actually harder in some ways, too. And let's be honest, I had such an amazing support crew. Family, friends, colleagues - even my hairdresser - were rooting for me! I can't really complain." - Mallory, 38

DOCTOR PERSPECTIVE: "It is a personal choice but, globally, it is recommended that you should tell as many people you are comfortable with telling. Any concern is often met with pleasant surprise." - Dr. Paul C. Lin, Seattle Reproductive Medicine, 2019-2020 SART President

Should I tell my family?

This is entirely up to you. It's generally advised to let people know what you're facing so they be there to support you and help out if you need, but this depends on your relationship with your family and your own personal preference. Be prepared that not everyone will approve of or support a decision to egg freeze because of their own beliefs, or they may have fears or reservations about the procedure out of concern for you. However, most of the time families are very supportive of the decision (especially future potential grandparents!)

"I feel like all my parents want is for me to find a husband and have kids so they can be grandparents. But this just isn't in the cards for me right now. I decided to freeze my eggs and wasn't going to tell them at all but changed my mind when I had to start taking the injections. I told my mom and she freaked out a bit, thinking that I'd basically thrown in the towel in motherhood. Once I talked through it, she became one of my biggest supporters. It's actually brought us so much closer." - Meg, 36

"I come from a conservative, religious family so I was absolutely dreading raising egg freezing with my parents - my dad in particular. After I told them, they stared at me with puzzled faces for what felt like a very long, very silent time, but once they wrapped their heads around it, they were actually pretty into it! My mom was so happy to know that I do actually want kids and my dad was relieved that I wouldn't feel obligated to marry just anyone because of my ticking biological clock (some of my friends have gotten divorced for this reason and they're very against it.)" - Trang, 32

"I literally don't know what I would have done if I hadn't told my parents. My mom cooked healthy meals during the three months prior. My dad picked me up after my procedure and both of my parents were there to help me recover. I feel really lucky to have them." - Beth, 30

"I tend to be pretty independent and I've never had a great relationship with my parents so telling them wasn't even a question. I have created my own family with my friends and they were more than supportive during the process." - Amelia, 38

Should I tell my friends?

It's normal to feel a bit unsure about how widely to discuss your egg freezing plans. You might be more naturally comfortable talking about this sort of thing, or not. And, not all your friends are alike. Some might be in a totally different place in their lives and egg freezing isn't something they've even thought about before. Or, another common scenario is that opening up the conversation with a friend will spark an, "OMG I've been thinking about it too!" reaction. On the other side of the spectrum, many women struggle in struggle in silence if they're dealing with infertility, so approaching the topic might be likely to bring up other feelings along the way.

"I am literally the ONLY one of my friends that is not married with babies - the token Bridget Jones of the group. I dropped the news that I was freezing my eggs at one of their kid's birthday parties. All I heard was crickets for what seemed like a lifetime. Once they processed what I was talking about they were so excited for me. It was so foreign to them at first but they totally rallied behind me throughout the whole process." - Izzy, 32

"I feel like egg freezing is the 'new norm' in my friend group. They really helped me navigate how I was feeling every step of the way. They even made me a recovery day survival kit with bone broth, magazines, and a facemask." - Rebecca, 38

"I was encouraged to freeze my eggs by a friend going through IVF. I've been there for her through her infertility struggle and she begged me to freeze my eggs so that I wouldn't end up in the same position she was. I felt a bit awkward about it at first because I had a good egg freezing outcome and didn't want to make her feel bad about her own situation but she was the exact opposite. It made me realize how important it is for all of us to be supporting each other during this weird fertility road that we're all on." - Charlotte, 34

Should I tell my partner? (Women's perspectives)

Again, this is entirely up to you. However, if you're in a long-term relationship or live together it would be advisable, given this is likely a decision that relates to both of your futures and you might want to lean on your partner for some support during the hormone injecting phase, or ask him or her to pick you up after the procedure. Most people don't know a great deal about fertility in general, let alone the nuances of egg freezing. Be prepared for some questions, puzzlement - even embarrassment. Remember just because someone doesn't fully understand, *doesn't* mean they're not willing to support you. Many women actually say they found egg freezing a great opportunity to talk to their partner about their reasons (buying some time, easing some pressure, health concerns) or larger relationship dynamics:

"This was one of the most challenging questions I had going into the procedure ... I had been dating my boyfriend for around a year and he was quite a bit younger than me. He was sweet and awesome, but he just didn't really have his life sorted out. Deep down I knew he was more of a 'Mr. Right Now' than 'Mr. Right.' I knew we'd have to part ways at some point, thanks mostly to our different life stages, but I just didn't feel like I wanted to bring up awkward conversations about eggs and ticking clocks when having a baby was so clearly not on his radar. Freezing my eggs actually woke me up to reality. Not long after, we had a sad, but really respectful, break up - we still keep in touch every now and then and he'll always be special to me." - Kacey, 37

"I had only been on a few dates with a guy when I decided to freeze my eggs. I was so conflicted about whether or not to tell him. I was really worried he would think I was trying to pressure him into fatherhood. So, rather than tell him outright, I asked him what he thought of other women freezing their eggs.. His exact response was, 'I think every woman should do it. It's fantastic!' Once I told him I was doing it, he was amazingly supportive throughout the procedure and it's actually been a positive milestone in our relationship (we're still together) - Chloe, 35

"I'd been seeing Mike for about six months and felt like, if I can't tell him about something medical...is he really the one for me anyway? He was completely cool about it, of course. We actually didn't end up staying together, but that had nothing to do with the fact I froze my eggs. It just didn't work out." - Veronica, 34

Should I tell my partner? (Men's perspectives)

Let's assume your partner is a guy and hear from some of them. (Not to generalize, but we're assuming female partners are likely more in the know!) Of course, not every man is going to have the same opinion on egg freezing. But out of the men we've spoken to – a range of single guys, boyfriends, fiancés, husbands, dads and even grandfathers, we have been bowled over by how the vast, vast majority of them are egg freezing fans.

"My girlfriend and I had been dating for about a year when she told me she was thinking about it. I honestly had no idea what she was talking about at first but once she explained it, I didn't see any downside. Now that she's done it, she just seems more chilled. It's been awesome for us." - Will, 33

"My ex-girlfriend did it and I was against it. I just don't think that you should mess with God's plan." - Jacob, 33

"I think it was only our second Tinder date when it came up in conversation that she was going to freeze her eggs. I wasn't sure what to say, but I thought it was kind of cool. I asked her if she minded me asking questions and then we chatted about it for a while. It didn't feel like a big deal, I just found it interesting and I respect her for doing it." - Marc, 34

"Egg freezing is f*cking awesome. I only date girls that have frozen their eggs, haha. They aren't trying to get married after our first date." - Brian, 37

ELANZA PERSPECTIVE: "There's sometimes a notion that women in their thirties and beyond are like hawks circling above an ever-dwindling field of men, ready to tuck their wings in and dive bomb one if he so much as glances in her direction. Guys often tell us that, contrary to this, they find the idea that a woman has frozen her eggs makes her seem self-assured, composed and practical. Strong, but kind of vulnerable, too - and that's attractive." - Brittany & Catherine

Should I tell my boss / co-workers?

There's no right or wrong answer to this and there's no legal requirement to, but it would likely make scheduling work around your appointments and procedure an easier process. Even where companies offer egg freezing as part of a benefits package, it should be a fairly anonymous process, like other healthcare perks:

"I didn't tell anyone at work and it was the most awkward experience ever. I was late a couple times because of the scans and needed to slip out of a fairly major meeting. I didn't know what to say other than 'I have a medical appointment.' We have open plan seating so everyone noticed and I'm sure there was all kinds of gossip. One day I even had to bring my cooler bag of meds with a pharmaceutical company logo into work. My advice would be to tell everyone at work up front. For me, it would have been far less stressful in the long run!" - Lisa, 35

"I told my boss because I wanted to make sure I didn't have any clashes with appointments, and, honestly, so he'd be less likely to give me a giant project that month. I just found it easier to be open about it. He was a bit neutral about it, like he wasn't sure how to react, but he eventually ended up suggesting that I work from home when I needed to, which was great." - Jo, 37

"I was able to work from home for a few days in the last bit of taking the injections when I was pretty bloated and then take a sick day for the actual procedure, thanks to my manager. I figured if I talked to my team about it, they'd probably be flexible and they really were. In fact, I'm so glad I told them as everyone was really sweet and sent encouraging messages!" - Heidi, 29

Should I talk to a professional?

If you do end up feeling particularly stressed or anxious during the treatment cycle, scientific evidence suggests that getting support from a trained professional can benefit your reproductive system. For example, Cognitive Behavior Therapy (CBT) and Neurolinguistic Programming (NLP), can reduce anxiety and stress in IVF patients, offer relief from negative thought spirals and possibly improve fertility function.[1539] [1540] [1541] [1542] [1543] [1544] [1545] [1546] [1547]

"My mom thought I should go to therapy as she'd heard lots of stories of people doing IVF and finding it tough. I think she was worried about the effect the meds were going to have on me and probably thought I was panicking about not having kids. But, to be honest, I'm not even sure I want them and I just wasn't that rocked by the whole thing. All the way along, I just felt like 'yep, I'm going to do it. It's a little scary, but let's just get it over with.' And even with the hormones, I carried on as usual at work and genuinely felt ok." - Tracy, 36

"Talking to a therapist wasn't something I'd ever considered, but after my friend suggested having a few sessions I gave it a shot. I was surprised how much pent up emotion I'd been carrying around in me about my divorce and how resentful I was having to freeze my eggs, all the while telling myself I was completely fine. My therapist ended up helping me in ways I didn't even know I'd needed." - Yasmin, 43

7. Create a positive mindset and routine

Don't underestimate the power of the mind/ovary connection, for better or for worse. Depressive symptoms and anxiety (and some coping mechanisms linked to them) are associated with lower rates of pregnancy.[1548] [1549] [1550] [1551] While this could be a case of correlation, not causality, some scientists think there could be hormonal effects at play. Daily disciplines that minimize your chance of experiencing these should be a real focus, for self-care as much as your egg freezing outcome.

There are a few simple activities you can add to your routine that have been shown to help people manage emotional turbulence. These simple activities are especially worth making time for during the stimulation cycle when the hormones are running high:

Start a journal

Even spending five minutes a day writing about your experience can help you organize your thoughts and regulate your emotions.[1552] Use this constructive "me time" as a mental space to document your hopes and fears and to explore questions about the future (especially now that you'll have your eggs on ice!).

If you struggle with an empty page, or if writing just isn't your thing, try using a prompt, like "Five Minute Journal" or "One Line Every Day" (both available on Amazon or bookstores), which help prompt and guide you. Or, simply write an email to a close friend if you find that an easier approach, even if you never send it.

"It was a relief to unload some of my thoughts and feelings onto the page about the long-term health problems I've faced. I don't know if it helped me make sense of them, but it definitely stopped me from bottling it all up so much and helped me to have more awareness around how I was really feeling, day-to-day." - Gabrielle, 27

Conscious breathing exercises

"I don't think I was mentally prepared for how I'd feel once I started taking the hormone injections. I was pretty emotional throughout. Doing really simple, conscious breathing exercises - like breathing in for five counts and out for seven counts - helped release some tension and settle my pulse, which felt like it was racing every time I started overthinking everything." - Sarah, 37

Meditation

"I really suck at meditation and all that kind of stuff. But I found putting on a podcast that guided me through it really helped me sit quietly, close my eyes and get into it. Twenty minutes at a time actually flew by and I really felt calmer and more focused after. When I meditated before work, I was less likely to bite the heads off of my co-workers, too." - Isabelle, 35

Calming yoga

"I heard yoga could help with stress as well as managing some of the physical side effects, but I couldn't actually afford classes after saving up literally every penny for months to do egg freezing. So I just put on pregnancy yoga online videos and made it work for me! It ended up being my favorite part of my day and I was really glad to have that space to just relax and feel like I was looking after myself." - Sunita, 40

Body scanning / "progressive muscle relaxation" (PMR)

"There's this technique called body scanning that I actually found insanely relaxing right before going to sleep when I was stressed. You basically lie down, close your eyes and relax one muscle at a time, starting from your toes and working up to your face in sequence, until your whole body is in a state of relaxation. It was so soothing that I'd forget what I was nervous or worried about and be asleep so much faster than when my mind was all over the place." - Olivia, 36

Pamper yourself

"I went to town with baths. I mean it! Like, every night, candles, music or a podcast and I soaked away my stress for as long as I felt like it. It felt great to not feel like I should be planning anything. I gave myself permission to just chill." - Zoe, 38

Rest and take care of yourself, but don't plan on doing <u>nothing</u>...

The hormone stimulation period is totally the time to give yourself a break from trying to run the world: get someone else to do the cooking, skip doing the laundry and don't feel the need to reply to all your messages straight away. Instead, give yourself a hall pass to put your feet up and watch a good movie, disconnect and read a book or indulge in a few treats. With that said, taking some injections each day really doesn't mean that you'll have to go into hiding. In fact, some healthy distractions at the right points might give you a positive lift.

DOCTOR PERSPECTIVE: "I recommend that my patients try to continue with their normal life and pursue what they usually like to do." - Dr. Paul C. Lin, Seattle Reproductive Medicine, 2019-2020 SART President

Key takeaways

- Before your treatment, set up your schedule for success.

- Plan out where and how you're going to get your prescriptions in advance (and potentially save some money and time by doing some due diligence beforehand!)

- Clear up any unknowns with your doctor before your treatment - it will give you better peace of mind.

- You can expect to follow the main lifestyle components from the rest of this guide but there are a few special things to consider over the stimulation phase, related to diet, exercise, supplements and more. Review them beforehand so you can be prepared to make those modifications to your lifestyle.

- There is no single answer to how you're going to feel emotionally.

- Making simple changes to prepare emotionally can prevent regrets, potentially improve the outcome and foster better decision making and clarity.

- Establish a support system - connect with other women, talk to family and friends and possibly your workplace or a professional counselor or therapist.

- Create a positive mindset routine using tools and techniques such as journaling, conscious breathing, meditation and yoga.

CHECKLIST: PRE-TREATMENT

☐ Adjust schedule to accommodate for potential time needed for clinic appointments, medication pickup, the retrieval procedure, and recovery

☐ Give colleagues a heads up that schedule might be different than normal

☐ Determine where you want to store your eggs

☐ Determine which pharmacy to get your medication from and how to get them

☐ If you don't feel comfortable doing the injections your self, get a friend or concierge nurse to do it for you

☐ Stock up on healthy snacks and easy-to-prepare meals

☐ Talk to the doctor about any supplements and/or medications you're currently taking

☐ Clear up any questions or unknowns with the doctor or clinic

☐ Establish a support system by talking to fellow freezers, friends, family, your partner, and/or co-workers

☐ Establish a positive mindset routine that you can carry out throughout your treatment.

A downloadable version of this checklist is available at ELANZAwellness.com.

Chapter 15: What to Expect Day-by-day Throughout Ovarian Stimulation

"Never bend your head. Always hold it high. Look the world straight in the eye."

- Helen Keller

No one can foresee exactly how the cycle is going to go down for you: every woman's egg freezing cycle follows a slightly different timeline, duration, and outcome. When you head into an egg freezing cycle, you're going to need to expect the unexpected to a certain degree. But, based on average cycles, here's our stimulation cycle roadmap, to give you an idea of what to expect at each stage and the landmarks to watch out for along the journey:

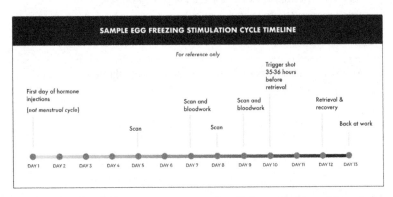

This timeline follows an average cycle of about 12 days, although the exact duration will depend on how your ovaries respond to the injections. If the cycle takes more of less time than this, it doesn't mean anything is wrong, it just means your ovaries are responding to the hormones at their own pace. Timing can be affected by age and medical conditions such as PCOS.

DAY 1: Injections begin

This is the first day you inject the fertility hormones. Exactly when you start your injections will depend on the treatment protocol prescribed by your doctor, which you need to follow precisely. During the first few days of injections, you most likely won't feel too affected by the hormones, physically or emotionally, but figuring out how to inject the hormones can be a bit intimidating.

Demystifying the medications

Many women say they get confused or worried about the medications. Here's a quick run through the main protocols of medications, which vary depending on whether your doctor anticipates you being a low, normal or high responder. Once your doctor gives you an indication on where you fit on this spectrum, they're likely to prescribe one of the protocols below, or some minor variation of them. Keep in mind that this is for explanation only and is not a substitute for your doctor's advice:

Normal and high responders: The gold standard is the Antagonist protocol, in which, in addition to stimulation medications (gonadotropins), "GnRH antagonist" drugs (common brands are Ganirelix or Cetrotide) are injected to shut off the surge of luteinizing hormone from your pituitary gland. This prevents ovulation *during* stimulation to make sure all the eggs will still be in your ovaries at egg retrieval. Less common is another type of protocol called the "long agonist" protocol, in which "GnRH agonists" (such as Lupron) are injected to prevent ovulation. This was the most common protocol prior to the development of GnRH antagonists. The disadvantage is you inject Lupron for two to three weeks, whereas GnRH antagonists typically only have to be injected for the final four to five days of the stimulation cycle.

Low responders: "Short agonist" - also called "flare" or "micro-dose" - agonist protocols involve starting agonist injections earlier than in the above, on around the first or second day of your period, followed the next day by the start of the gonadotropins. This protocol is designed to stimulate your body's own FSH production, followed by stimulation with gonadotropins (FSH) to maximize stimulation and maturation of eggs. By about one week into the stimulation, the GnRH agonist, just as in the Long Agonist protocol, inhibits ovulation. Normal or high responders do not need to have their own FSH stimulated, so may over-respond to this protocol.

In all cycles women also inject a "trigger shot", to re-expose the mature eggs to luteinizing hormone (LH) prior to egg retrieval. Read more about this crucial shot in the "trigger shot" section.

"On the first day of shots, my mind completely blanked and I couldn't remember what the nurse told me about how to inject the medications… I was so embarrassed to have to call them to ask to run through it again, but I felt so much better when I did" - Liz, 27

"I was worried about the injections at first but after I did it once, it just became part of my daily routine." - Fran 39

"I really didn't think I had a problem with needles... until I had to administer the shots myself. Everyone says that it's almost the same exact thing that diabetics have to inject every day, so I figured it couldn't be too bad. But when I tried it myself, I thought I'd done it incorrectly and then nearly fainted. Maybe it was a low blood sugar thing. It was all fine eventually. I actually asked my coworker to help me with the injections each morning!" - Tanya, 32

ELANZA INSIGHT: "We found the best way to do the injections was to get it all lined up and ready to go, then take a long, deep inhale...as you exhale, gently slide the needle in to your squished up belly fat. Don't be in a panic to get it over with in a split second. There is zero need to rush, and doing it in time with your breath can help you stay calm, feel in control and genuinely makes it pretty painless." - Brittany and Catherine

DAYS 2 - 6

At this stage, you could start to feel some effects of PMS, both physical and emotional. Many women say the emotional sensitivity during the second half of the stimulation cycle is like an enhanced version of their usual symptoms of PMS. On the other hand, many women don't report having any emotional fluctuations at all! In fact, some of them reported having positive emotions that highlighted their own feelings of relief and empowerment afforded by the procedure itself.

You might also notice some minor bruising on your abdomen from the needle but that's quite normal. If it bothers you, doctors often advise simply moving the injection site a tiny bit from one day to the next as not to aggravate the area.

You'll likely go into the clinic for one or more scans to see how your ovaries are responding to the injections. During the scan your doctor will be able to show you on the monitor what your follicles look like inside your ovaries (they show up like small black circles on the screen). The doctor will be able to measure a few of them to see how they're progressing, and he or she will most likely be able to give you a rough count on how many are growing.

It's important to note that not all of the follicles will yield an egg (some doctors say this is because it's hard to tell the difference between a cyst and a follicle). And not all the follicles retrieved at the end of the cycle will be mature enough to yield a mature egg (typically a follicle needs to measure at least 14-15mm in order to produce a mature egg worth freezing). So while it's a key metric for your doctor to keep track of in order to know how much medication to prescribe you and how long the cycle should be (possibly even to try to "predict" how many eggs you will retrieve), try not to get too caught up on how many follicles you have. Ovarian stimulation is not an exact science. Some would even call it an "ART"...

"I really didn't start to feel any real differences for the first week of injections. I did get some bruising on my stomach and started to feel a little bloating it wasn't until around the trigger shot that I felt more tired than usual." - Belinda, 33

"I'm about a week in and I'm starting to feel kind of over it. My energy is low, I'm cranky and my tummy has some bruising from the injections, which isn't a big deal, but also isn't fun." - Jolize, 37

DAYS 7 - 9

Some women report very uncomfortable abdominal bloating, while others don't notice much of a change. The advice is to keep drinking lots of fluids and to take it easy - no extreme or high impact exercise and/or twisting motions.

"My bloating wasn't bad in the morning, but in the afternoon I was a bit uncomfortable. I chose a loose dress with a tie around the waist so I could loosen it as needed. I hit a bit of a wall around 4-5pm and started to feel pretty tired and cranky (as I have for the last few days)." - Kerry, 36

"I have to pee CONSTANTLY. It feels like being pregnant! How ironic." - Mel, 38

"Surprisingly, I'm less bloated than the day before but my ovaries feel heavy. It's been really uncomfortable to sleep so I feel tired, which isn't helping with the overall blah feeling. I went to a yin yoga class though and it was fine." - Jessie, 37

DAY 10: The "trigger shot"

When your doctor thinks your follicles are mature enough, she or he will advise you to stop taking your fertility medication and administer a "trigger" shot of hormones. Because ovulation needs to be "turned off" (using either GnRH agonists or antagonists, as explained earlier in this chapter), it is important to re-expose the mature eggs to Luteinizing Hormone (LH) prior to the egg retrieval. Remember that if the eggs do not get "triggered" with LH, or the analog of LH, hCG, the eggs will either not come out of the ovaries upon aspiration of the follicles (sometimes called "empty follicle syndrome," a misnomer because the follicles aren't empty, the eggs just remain stuck in the follicles and don't come out), or the eggs that do come out are immature.

With the trigger injection, timing is everything. It is typically injected exactly 36 hours prior to the egg retrieval, when the eggs will still be there. If the egg retrieval were to be delayed to 39+ hours after the trigger injection, the eggs would likely have been ovulated into the pelvis and therefore, not retrievable.

For women on the GnRH antagonist protocol, an alternative trigger to hCG is to administer Lupron 36 hours prior to egg retrieval. This causes a woman's own pituitary LH to be released – the LH surge. Because LH is a rapidly metabolized hormone, it is cleared from the body relatively quickly, as compared to hCG which lingers for as much as week and can continue to stimulate the ovarian follicles after the egg retrieval. This puts high responders at risk of ovarian hyperstimulation syndrome.

DOCTOR PERSPECTIVE: "For high responders, we commonly use 1/10th the dose of hCG used for normal or low responders, in conjunction with a Lupron trigger to mature the eggs. However, one group of high responders cannot use Lupron triggers - women with hypothalamic anovulation (runners, gymnasts, ballet dancers, let's say, who have very low body fat and no ovulation). In these women, the pituitary does not make LH so a Lupron trigger is ineffective." - Dr. Carolyn Givens, Pacific Fertility Center, San Francisco

Luckily your doctor will be managing your medications and you simply need to administer it. Basically, what you need to know and focus on is that the *timing* of the trigger shot is arguably the most important part of the cycle. If you miss the time, it can significantly compromise the outcome of the entire cycle. So set an alarm, especially as it is often needs to be injected late in the evening, and consider having someone primed to remind you, as a backup. Review the instructions you've been given by your clinic about when exactly to take the remaining shots.

"I went in for my third scan and had my last shots of the stimulation medications. The doctor seems to think that I'm coming along well, with the largest of my follicles being about 25mm. My ovaries also look like they're overlapping with one another. The doctor said they tend to move closer together as the follicles get larger, which was more likely to happen because I have PCOS." - Katy, 32

"I've been going to work everyday but when I get home all feel like doing is lying down horizontally and watching TV." - Britta, 35

"I haven't felt particularly uncomfortable. I think I've just been lucky. But after taking the trigger shot, I've definitely noticed more bloating. It feels like bad gas! I'm restless and can't get comfortable. I've been really relaxed the whole way through and now right at the last hurdle it's really hitting me and I've started to feel like I just want the retrieval to happen already. I'd like my normal life back." - Angela, 37

DAY 11: Retrieval day preparation

Once your doctor schedules your retrieval procedure, there are a few things you'll want to do ahead of time:

- Remind the friend or family member who will be collecting you from the clinic of the place and time. Remember, in the US, you are not legally allowed to leave without being accompanied by a responsible adult.

- Review the instructions you've been given by your clinic about when exactly to take the remaining shots and other important considerations. It's very important that you avoid eating or drinking anything for eight hours or so prior to the egg retrieval. If you forget this, it is highly likely that the clinic will have to cancel your procedure.

- Pre-prepare some food for the next few days or have a food delivery service at the ready. You might not feel like cooking or grocery shopping during the day of your retrieval or even for a few days afterward.

- Download some good movies and podcasts, get some magazines, and think of this as a little staycation.

- Plan to spend the evening before relaxing and doing something that makes you feel your most serene and comfortable – maybe you light some candles and listen to your favorite music while doing a face mask, or simply watch an old movie that makes you laugh. Think: gentle distractions. Some breathing exercises or meditation might slow your pulse and dispel worries, if you find yourself struggling to get to sleep.

- It's very important that you avoid eating or drinking anything for eight hours or so prior to the egg retrieval. If you forget this, it is highly likely that the clinic will have to cancel your procedure. You would then have to start the process all over, including making up all the costs up to that point.

- When you arrive at the clinic on your retrieval day, they will have you fill out a form with questions about what you want to happen to your eggs in case something were to happen to you. As one can imagine, this can be a lot to take in… so it's worth taking the time beforehand to consider your options. Generally, you can choose one of the following: (a) give them away for research purposes like stem cell research, which would not result in the birth of a child; (b) to destroy the eggs; or (c) to donate the eggs to another or individual for reproductive purposes. In the US, if you choose this last option, you will need to pay extra for those eggs to undergo FDA screening and you will most likely need to name the person you'd like them to be donated to.

CHECKLIST: RETRIEVAL DAY PREP

- ☐ Confirm who is going to pick you up from the clinic and take you home after your retrieval
- ☐ **Adhere to the instructions given by the clinic** This includes the exact timing for your trigger shot and food and drink allowances before treatment
- ☐ Prepare some rejuvenating food for recovery (or have a food delivery service at the ready)
- ☐ Download some good movies and podcasts or buy some magazines
- ☐ Decide how you want your eggs to be treated in case anything were to happen to you
  Your options are:
  1. To give them away for research purposes like stem cell research, which would not result in the birth of a child
  2. To have them destroyed
  3. To donate the eggs to another or individual for reproductive purposes. (In the US, if you choose this option, you will need to pay extra for those eggs to undergo FDA screening and you will most likely need to name the person you'd like them to be donated to.

A downloadable version of this checklist is available at ELANZAwellness.com.

DAY 12: Retrieval day!

If you feel a bit anxious before the procedure, don't worry, that's totally normal. How it all happens depends on your clinic and doctor. But, here's a typical sequence of events:

When you arrive at the clinic, you'll get into a robe and be given a hospital bed. This is when you'll have to fill in the paperwork about what you want to happen to your eggs if something bad were to happen to you. Then, you'll be wheeled into the operating room where an anesthesiologist will gently put you to sleep. Your surgeon will retrieve your eggs by using ultrasound to help him or her carefully guide a fine, transvaginal needle through your vaginal wall into your ovaries, each in turn. The needle is attached to a tiny vacuum, which sucks out the follicle fluid containing the eggs. Once they've been removed, they'll be placed in the care of an embryologist in the lab, who will examine them and use liquid nitrogen to freeze them. Once the mature eggs have been identified, the embryologist will place your eggs on "straws" and dip the straws into tanks filled with liquid nitrogen.

"When I woke up I felt the bloating was at max discomfort. I couldn't wait to get to the clinic and actually have the procedure done." - Annika, 36

"I was so over it by the retrieval day. I just kept thinking 'get these things out of me!' I didn't even think about the surgery itself until right before, then I got a bit nervous." - Melissa, 38

"I felt quite calm. I'd spoken a lot to my doctor about what would be happening and I just wanted to try to stay Zen and not entertain all the racing questions like how many eggs I'd get and how quickly I'd feel back to normal. My Mom dropped me off, but I didn't have her come in with me as I didn't want to talk, I preferred to tune out. I listened to an audiobook until the last possible moment." - Juliana, 37

You'll wake up in the recovery room roughly 15-20 minutes after you were first put to sleep – it will feel like you've just woken up from the world's biggest nap. Once the nurse thinks you are well enough, you can get dressed and go home. Your doctor's advice will almost certainly be to rest for the remainder of the day. If you're like most women, you will be groggy and feel more like curling up in bed or on the sofa and sleeping it off, rather than heading into the office. Very occasionally, someone may have a reaction to the sedative – in that case, the medical team will treat you accordingly. If you feel faint or sick, you may be given a drip to help you recover. You'll be notified either that day or the next on the total number of mature eggs they were able to retrieve and freeze.

"The team was so nice when I came around after the retrieval. One of the nurses gave me a piece of paper with the number of eggs they got written on it. I was actually disappointed as I got 5 eggs and was hoping for more, but they were really great about it and I think that's what made it easier to handle." - Mia, 37

"I spent pretty much all day in bed. It was hard to stand upright without feeling like my uterus was going to fall out. This is definitely TMI, but I had the runs, as well as the feeling when you're really gassy and it feels trapped inside you. I was able to eat a little bit but would feel queasy. It was like the worst PMS ever." - Priya, 37

"I didn't feel too bad. The awful bloated feeling went away quite soon after the procedure. But I was just so exhausted I slept the whole afternoon. I only got up in the evening to have something to eat, but I hardly felt like it." - Jess, 35

DAY 13+: Recovery

The majority of women are able to go back to work the next day. On the other hand, it could take four or five days for the discomfort and bloating to fully go away. Luckily, there's a time limit to the annoying symptoms - you'll feel yourself getting more back to normal each day. It takes a while for your body to get rid of the extra hormones and for your ovaries to settle back to their natural state.

With that said, this is the time that you should remain aware of any signs and symptoms of OHSS and flag anything considered abnormal. Remember, the warning signs of OHSS are: abdominal pain, severe bloating, nausea, vomiting, diarrhea, tenderness in ovaries area and sudden weight increase (water retention). If you are in pain, or you suspect you might have OHSS, phone the emergency number or follow the procedure your clinic advises. It's always worth flagging concerns with your medical team, who can best advise you.

If all has gone broadly to plan, no other scans or medical tests are needed. Your clinic will be able to tell you the number of eggs frozen and their maturity. Depending on the number of eggs obtained, you may want to follow-up with the clinic to discuss whether or not you should do another cycle.

Women tell us they had these questions after their procedure was over:

When can I get back into my exercise routine?

Immediately following the procedure, you'll probably feel groggy and physically uncomfortable as the sedative wears off, so physical activity won't likely sound appealing nor is it a good idea. A few days to a week after your retrieval surgery, your abdomen might still be bloated and sensitive as your ovaries will still be enlarged. During this time, you might be at risk of ovarian torsion, so most doctors advise women to wait for at least ten to twelve days before taking any strenuous activity to let the body reset. Keeping generally active, such as with gentle walking, will help eliminate retained fluid. Some doctors also say to avoid swimming or being submerged in water right before and for at least twelve days after your ovarian stimulation, as it could expose your retrieval site to bacteria and infections. Plus, the effects of chlorine on your reproductive system are unknown.

When will my next period start?

Your cycle should return to normal the month after the procedure, though there are exceptions to this, especially if you usually have rare or irregular periods. Spotting can occur any time after the retrieval, and your period should arrive somewhere around ten to twelve days following the procedure. If your cycle does not start within two weeks of the procedure, let your clinic know.

How soon can I have sex?

Don't have sex for at least ten to twelve days after retrieval in order to give yourself enough time to heal and to decrease the risk of infection. And (broken record here) don't forget birth control! You could be mega fertile!

Chapter 17: The Future - "What Should I do Now?"

"Life can only be understood backwards; but it must be lived forwards."

— Søren Kierkegaard

You did it! Now what? Let's talk about the really hard thing that nobody seems to cover: what comes next.

If you got the result you wanted

Even if everything goes to plan and a satisfactory number of eggs were retrieved, some women have admitted they felt a bit "empty" or "unsure what to do next" once the cycle was over. It's not like anything else really changes. When an event has been on the horizon for a long time, particularly something that feels like the solution to a problem, and then the event passes, it can leave you feeling a bit adrift and without a clear practical focus. That's perfectly normal. It's kind of like how some brides get depressed after their weddings: without all the planning, without the nerves and the preparation, without a role to play.

OK, here's the thing. You're you. And always will be. Ultimately, egg freezing isn't going to glow you up into a different woman, magic up a perfect partner (well, unless you subscribe to our highly speculative "egg freezing as cupid" theory!) or transform your problems away. Just like if you leave home for vacation feeling flat, frustrated or unhappy with life, and when you get there you wake up with the same feelings creeping in after a couple of days when the novelty wears off. You took "you" with you, as they say.

"Egg freezing didn't change anything. I mean, I don't think I was expecting it to, but it was still strange to think here I am, still no boyfriend, still unhappy in my job, still no idea when I'm going to be ready to be at the kind of stage all my friends are at. I'm glad and grateful I stored 11 eggs, I know that's really good for my age. But, it still feels depressing that I might need to use them." – Carla, 37

The crucial difference is that you have eggs on ice, and that's all this procedure set out to do. We can all get caught up in words like "transformational" and "empowering" and "life-changing" and fall victim to the promise of the marketing materials featuring photographs of laughing women in extremely together outfits, looking like they are absolutely owning it (whatever "it" is). But, in reality, you might not feel like that right after.

You head home, sleep it off, get up and carry on with your life. Which stills looks exactly like your life, except you've now completed your egg freezing cycle. Getting back to just being you can be a great thing. But if that's not a good feeling, if that's the thing that needs the change, then there's the answer of what you can do next. Change. Grow. Figure out what's not working for you in your life and make that your next project. All this is your own, personal show and you get to call the shots.

"As soon as I recovered, I went back to work and really just forgot about it. I know I've got time, especially with my eggs saved, so I try not to think about it too much. I am dating, but mostly I'm focused on work. I know where I want to be in three to five years in my life and I think that will happen. I tell all my girlfriends to freeze their eggs, why not make contingency plans?" – Vasundera, 33

"I did three rounds of freezing, so I feel good about the number of eggs I have stored. But, I don't have a partner and it feels like every man I meet is happily married, going through a horrendous divorce or gay. It wouldn't be my first choice to have a baby by myself, even though the financial side of things wouldn't be a problem. But who knows, maybe in two or three years if I still haven't met anyone, then I'll choose that route. I'm pretty realistic about my fertility." – Maura, 40

If the results weren't what you wanted...

There's no sugarcoating it, this can be a very low, frustrating time - even full on devastating - if fewer eggs were retrieved than you were hoping for.

"It felt like my body had failed me and I had failed at a test run of motherhood. It took a lot of conversations and reflections for me to make peace with it and feel ok again." - Francesca, 40

It's perfectly ok to experience a low period afterwards. There's no getting around the fact that it would have been better had things gone another way. But, after you've given yourself time to get mad at the world and process your feelings however you do that best, take some time to reflect on these things:

Having a relatively low number of eggs retrieved does not necessarily equate to lower fertility. Researchers have found there is actually no correlation between ovarian reserve and your ability to get pregnant.[1553] So if you have a diminished ovarian reserve, low AMH measurement, or high FSH — you are no less likely to get pregnant than women with a normal AMH level. So, although AMH is a great way to predict egg yield in an ovarian stimulation cycle, it's not a good biomarker for actual conception.[1554 1555 1556] Women with low ovarian reserves may conceive *naturally* without issue.

DOCTOR INSIGHT: "A low number of eggs retrieved does NOT equate to lower fertility. That's because we predict fertility by egg quality, not quantity." - Dr. Meera Shah, Nova IVF, Mountain View

While the number of eggs frozen does affect the chance those eggs could one day result in a healthy baby, don't forget that ultimately what's needed to make a baby is *one* good quality egg. Lots of women still conceive naturally in their late 30s and even early 40s, it just might take longer for you. Getting pregnant depends on a lot of different complicated factors — not just how many eggs are left in your ovaries.

DOCTOR INSIGHT: "For my patients that have only had a few eggs retrieved, I remind them that all it takes is a single egg to make a baby. For example, I just thawed an egg from a patient whose eggs I froze about five years ago. It survived and tomorrow I'll find out if it's a blastocyst!" - Dr. Aimee Eyvazzadeh, Private Practice Physician, San Ramon

- If this was your first egg freezing cycle, ask your doctor what could be done differently for a subsequent cycle. The treatment protocol is often adjusted for known "poor responders" to ovarian stimulation, which can mean better results on another cycle.

- You have solid metrics now, whereas if you'd never done the cycle, you wouldn't have as much data to work this. Could this outcome make you make different decisions - like whether to try to have kids sooner? Results can be clarifying and that's a good thing, but remember to base any decisions on concrete interpretations from your doctor.

Don't struggle on your own. Your doctor is there to have an open and transparent discussion after the cycle, and beyond.

Do I need another cycle?

Lots of women do two or three rounds of egg freezing to get a "recommended" number of eggs on ice. If your doctor finds there weren't a sufficient number of mature eggs from your cycle, she or he may suggest another round, or perhaps you have a "minimum number of eggs" or multi-round package. This is something to weigh financially, emotionally and practically. Remember that you are under no obligation to use the same doctor and clinic. You may want to explore package deals that are based on delivering a minimum number of eggs regardless of the number of cycles needed to achieve that number, rather than paying per cycle. Check the chart below to see how many eggs you would need to store to get a good (75%) chance of them making a baby:

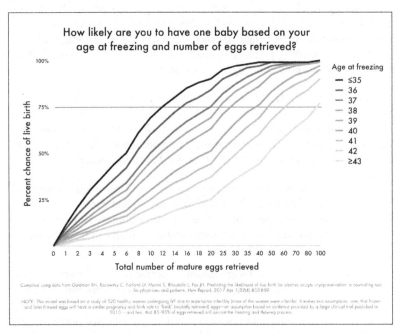

The numbers can feel overwhelming, especially if you didn't get many eggs retrieved on the first cycle. Bring this knowledge with you during your conversation with your doctor about whether a subsequent cycle is a good course of action. And, remember, the goal is always natural conception. Your frozen eggs are just a back-up.

EXPERT PERSPECTIVE: "I personally did three cycles and went to three different fertility clinics. I chose a different fertility center each cycle of my freezes to not put all my eggs in one basket. I had a great experience each time and with each group." - Valerie Landis, Fertility Patient Advocate

How soon can I do another cycle?

You can start the process again once your natural period returns. It might depend on how quickly your ovaries recover.

DOCTOR PERSPECTIVE: "Some studies suggest you get more and better eggs with back-to-back cycles. I think the data is mixed so I generally leave it up to how the patient is feeling. If they feel up to it I will put them on an oral contraceptive for a few weeks to give their ovaries some time to heal and then go back to a stimulation about three weeks after the last retrieval. I actually think there is some benefit to doing that. Again if the theory of the assembly line of developing follicles is correct then you may be able to get some benefit from piggybacking on a prior stimulation cycle that may result in higher number of eggs recruited in a subsequent cycle." - Dr. Diana Chavkin, HRC Fertility, Los Angeles

DOCTOR PERSPECTIVE: "We sometimes recommend a 'rest cycle' to allow the ovaries to heal and the person to feel completely back to normal before doing it again." - Dr. Meera Shah, Nova IVF, Mountain View

Ongoing storage of your eggs

Depending on your agreement with the clinic, you will either pay an annual fee for storage, or you will have a certain period of time covered as part of the cycle cost. Make sure to check when the first payment is due and set a calendar reminder. Generally, the clinic/storage facility will send an invoice for the upcoming storage fee. Just make sure they have your most up-to-date email address and billing information on file in case it changes or if your credit card expires. Your eggs should remain in situ for as long you pay the storage fees. Most practices have a time period if you "abandon" them, i.e. do not communicate or pay storage fees - at that point they will move forward with discarding them. Read the fine print. The typical duration is five years from last contact. Remember that in some countries such as the UK and Sweden, there are limitations on how long you can store frozen eggs, though these outdated rules are being challenged.

If you want to use your eggs in the future and do IVF at a different clinic, or if you move and wish to store them closer to your home, it's possible to transport your eggs. There is no evidence to suggest this will harm them, although of course there are small risks involved as there are when moving and transporting anything. The cryotank in which your eggs are stored can stay frozen for around a week, so specialist couriers are able to transport them, even between countries (with the correct paperwork).

DOCTOR PERSPECTIVE: "Sometimes I tell my patients to split the eggs into two shipments in order to mitigate the risk of loss. This is especially true at the point where they may be having them transported from storage back to a clinic to create embryos, i.e. when the patient is older and cannot replace them." - Dr. Carolyn Givens, Pacific Fertility Center, San Francisco

Using your frozen eggs: if you struggle to conceive naturally

Using your frozen eggs is a decision made in conjunction with a fertility doctor - this could be the same doctor who you saw for egg freezing, but needn't be. Using your frozen eggs involves the standard protocol for IVF, except you'd get to skip the ovarian stimulation phase of treatment, as your egg freezing cycle was essentially the first third of an IVF cycle. The average cost of a cycle of IVF in the US is currently around $12,000, though it could be up to $20K. If you use a surrogate carrier, there would be an additional cost. Here is a general rundown about what the remaining two-thirds of the process entails:

- **Testing** - Blood tests and ultrasounds would be done on both you and your partner (unless you are using donor sperm) to confirm that you can move forward with treatment.

- **Egg thawing** - If you have a committed "sperm source" (that phrase again!) then all of your frozen eggs would be thawed at once in a lab by a specially trained lab technician called an embryologist. They are not usually thawed one at a time - this approach would be more expensive.

- **Fertilization via ICSI** - Your partner or donor sperm would then be used to fertilize your thawed eggs using a technique called intracytoplasmic sperm injection (ICSI). This technique requires an embryologist to select a single sperm and inject it directly into each one of your eggs. This process is almost always used when previously frozen eggs are being fertilized because the eggs can slightly harden after freezing, making it a bit more difficult for sperm to penetrate and fertilize as easily as they would with non-frozen eggs.

- **Embryo** - Next, the fertilized eggs would be cultured or "grown" in a laboratory, just as they might naturally within the womb. Some of the more advanced labs are able to grow these embryos to a more advanced stage known as a "blastocyst." Not all embryos will make it this far, but if they do, they're thought to be far more likely to lead to a live birth.[1557]

- **Genetic testing** - As we've discussed earlier in the book, at an additional cost, you have the option of having your embryos tested for chromosomal abnormalities, something called PGS (pre-implantation genetic screening). This is meant to sieve out any lower quality embryos that are less likely to lead to a successful birth.

- **Embryo transfer** - One, or occasionally two, of the resulting embryos would be transferred into the uterus at one time in the hope it results in a pregnancy. If any embryos are not used, they can be frozen and used again (if the initial embryo transfer did not result in pregnancy, or for future attempts).

Depending on your age, how many children you want and if the results of your future AMH test and antral follicle count scan suggest you are still ovulating healthy eggs, your doctor may suggest you try IVF with a fresh cycle of eggs (i.e. do another round of ovarian stimulation at that age). If you plan on using the same sperm source with all of those eggs, doctors often recommend combining both your fresh and frozen eggs together - doing the embryo culturing and any genetic testing - all at the same time. To do it separately would almost double the cost.

Looking forward: fertility treatments are improving by the day

If you're freezing your eggs now, or will be in the near future, it's probably going to be at least a few years before you'd go back to use them, if you end up doing so. The field of fertility is fast evolving, with technological tweaks happening each year that improve procedures and help doctors and scientists get better at what they are all working towards: improving your chances of having a baby.

Scientists are hard at work studying ovarian aging. And it's not hard to see why: as humans are living longer, the long-term health consequences of ovarian aging are becoming more and more significant. That's because our ovaries can have far-reaching clinical and psychological consequences on our health. Ovarian function affects everything from our metabolisms, hearts, brains, bones, responses to stress, likelihood of some cancers and mortality. As a result, poor reproductive health can act as the proverbial canary in a coal mine, signaling chronic diseases: reproductive problems can indicate the presence or likelihood of developing a host of illnesses.[1558]

Looking forward, there are also exciting things being studied - some near term and plausibly in use in the years to come, some still far off and theoretical – that could represent a significant expansion of options for women. These could include for instance, techniques to take follicles straight from the ovaries and mature human eggs in the lab, or laser treatments that could help improve egg health. These possible new techniques have the potential to transform how fertility treatments are administered, and even what we think of as the limitations of female fertility!

EXPERT PERSPECTIVE: "One of the issues with egg freezing at the moment is the need for two weeks of hormone injections to stimulate the ovaries. Future developments may include simplifying that. Retrieving immature eggs and completing their maturation in the lab might make an egg freezing cycle a lot easier to do." - Professor Richard Anderson, University of Edinburgh MRC Centre for Reproductive Health

EXPERT PERSPECTIVE: "Over the next ten years you can expect assisted reproduction to become more standardized, more automated, and more data driven. This combination should drive the cost to consumers down, make it easier to isolate and improve the steps that are keeping the pregnancy rates per embryo from rising even higher than they are today, and make IVF, proactive fertility management and prevention of genetic disease much more accessible than they are today." - Dr. David Sable, Healthcare and Life Science Investor

But while some on-the-cusp innovations could become part of everyday medicine soon enough for us to see the benefits, many of the things scientists are studying may never come to fruition in our lifetimes. As such, in addition to freezing your eggs, it's imperative that you protect your future options by taking every aspect of your reproductive health seriously now.

What else can you do?

We truly hope that you and your eggs will benefit from the research and perspectives included in this book. It's our ongoing mission to improve the experiences and the outcomes of egg freezing. Once you've been through the egg freezing experience, we would be grateful if you would consider sharing your reflections with us (this can be anonymous) so we can help clinics improve services for future patients. To do this, visit: www.elanzawellness.com/whole-patient-pledge and click "share your story" or simply scan this QR code:

If you found this book useful, you can also help others find it by leaving a review online at Amazon. For more tools, resources, stories and research, join our newsletter, visit our website and follow us on Instagram - @elanzawellness.

Writing this guide has been a labor of love that was sparked by our own challenges with treatment. We hope that we've played some role in helping you feel more informed, empowered, and prepared as you endeavor down your own fertility journey.

Made in the USA
Monee, IL
07 November 2023

45968099R00164